Clinical Pharmacology

Clinical Pharmacology

Paul Turner
M.D., B.Sc., F.R.C.P.
Professor of Clinical Pharmacology,
St Bartholomew's Hospital, London

Alan Richens
M.B., Ph.D., F.R.C.P.
Professor of Pharmacology and Materia Medica,
Welsh National School of Medicine, Cardiff

FOURTH EDITION

CHURCHILL LIVINGSTONE
EDINBURGH LONDON MELBOURNE AND NEW YORK 1982

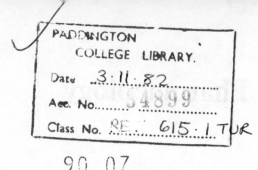
CHURCHILL LIVINGSTONE
Medical Division of Longman Group Limited

Distributed in the United States of America by
Longman Inc., 19 West 44th Street, New York,
N.Y. 10036 and by associated companies, branches and
representatives throughout the world.

First edition 1973
Second edition 1975
Third edition 1978
Fourth edition 1982

ISBN 0 443 02531 2

British Library Cataloguing in Publication Data

Turner, Paul
  Clinical pharmacology — 4th ed.
  1. Drugs 2. Pharmacology
  I. Title II. Richens, Alan
  615'.1   RM300

Library of Congress Catalog Card Number 81–67932

Printed in Singapore by
Huntsmen Offset Printing Pte Ltd.

Preface to the 4th Edition

Since our last revision the pharmacological basis of thrombosis, and particularly the importance of prostaglandins, prostacyclin and platelet function in that process, has received a great deal of attention. We have, therefore, devoted a chapter to the subject in this new edition, while carrying out a thorough revision of the whole book.

1982   P.T.
                                                                        A.R.

Contents

1

The assessment of new drugs

Until about one hundred years ago, most drugs used in the treatment of disease were derived from naturally-occurring substances of plant or animal origin, for example opium from the poppy, quinine from the cinchona tree and digitalis from the foxglove. In 1827 the glycoside salicin was extracted from the willow bark and in 1874 sodium salicylate was synthesized by Kolbe, introducing the era of synthetic therapeutics. Today the large majority of new therapeutic substances are synthesized in pharmaceutical laboratories and only few are obtained from natural sources.

Synthesis and screening
The development of a new drug occurs in the laboratories of a *synthetic chemist*, and is usually determined by structure activity considerations of related compounds. Sometimes, however, completely novel compounds are synthesized in order to evaluate their possible therapeutic effects. Following synthesis, the structure of the new compound and its purity are confirmed by an *analytical chemist*. It then passes to animal *pharmacologists* who screen (a) its pharmacological and (b) its toxic effects. The pharmacological studies are carried out by routine procedures in isolated organ preparations and in whole animals of different species. These are designed to detect significant activity in one or more systems of the body and to indicate possible mechanisms of action. Care has to be exercised to ensure that preparation of an animal for the experiment does not mask important pharmacological effects. For example, the neuromuscular-blocking activity of suxamethonium (succinyl choline) was missed in early experiments in which its possible ganglion-blocking action was studied in animals paralysed with curare.

Toxicological studies are carried out with both acute and chronic administration of the drug in varying doses. Acute studies show the doses necessary to kill a certain proportion of animals (e.g. LD_{50}) and the mode of death which occurs. Chronic studies are designed to detect the effects of its long-term administration over a major proportion of the animal's expected life span. Throughout both types of study close observation of the behaviour and physiological activities of the animals is carried out, as well as detailed biochemical and haematological measurements. After death careful histopathological examination of all tissues shows the effects of the drug on various body organs. It is evident that similar studies must be carried out at each stage on untreated control animals to determine which apparent abnormalities are due to the drug and which are associated with other inherited or environmental factors to which the animals are exposed.

Another group of toxicological studies which must be carried out on all new drugs is concerned with effects on reproduction. These assumed especial importance after recognition of the harmful effects of thalidomide on the developing foetus. These tests can be considered under three headings:

(a) Tests of fertility and general reproductive performance in which animals, usually rats, are treated with the new drug before and after mating and its influence on fertility in both sexes, the course of gestation, early and late stages of embryonic and foetal development, lactation and postnatal effects are studied.

(b) Teratological studies in which the effects of the drug on organogenesis are assessed. At least two species are used and the drug is given after mating during the period of organogenesis. Foetuses are carefully examined for visceral and skeletal abnormalities, the number of live and dead foetuses are recorded, and resorption sites in the uteri and the corpora lutea are examined and recorded.

(c) Adverse effects on the mother and offspring in the perinatal and postnatal stages are carried out by treatment during the last third of pregnancy and up to the period of weaning. Observations are made for delayed or prolonged labour, lactation, maternal care and direct toxic action of the drug on the young.

Once again, in all these tests, control groups of untreated animals have to be studied in sufficient numbers in order that the effects of the drug may be accurately assessed.

Biochemical studies

If preliminary screening measures indicate that the new compound has promising features, biochemical studies are carried out in experimental animals to determine its absorption by different routes of administration, its distribution throughout body compartments and its route of metabolism. If possible the blood and tissue levels required to produce pharmacological and toxic effects are determined. These investigations are often linked to pharmaceutical studies in which the effects of altering physical and physicochemical characteristics of the drug on its absorption are assessed. Such studies depend on the development of sensitive assay procedures involving gas–liquid chromatography, spectrophotofluorimetry, or radio-isotope techniques.

Before administering the new drug to man, it is becoming accepted practice in many countries to submit the information obtained from these pharmacological and biochemical studies to an independent government-appointed committee (e.g. the Committee on Safety of Medicines in Great Britain and the Food and Drug Administration in the United States of America). When approval has been given by this body, the drug may be administered to man.

Studies in man

Drug trials in man may be classified as (a) prophylactic, where a compound's ability to protect against disease is studied, for example, amantadine protecting against some forms of influenza, (b) therapeutic, in which the ability of a drug to treat a disease process already established is assessed, and (c) toxicological, where the emphasis of the investigation is on a drug's toxic rather than therapeutic effects. For example, although digitalis and aspirin have been in therapeutic use for many years, careful studies of the incidence and mechanism of their toxicity are still in progress. This discussion will be limited primarily to therapeutic clinical trials, and these may be subdivided further into (1) the pilot trial and (2) controlled trials.

The pilot trial

The pilot trial of a new drug is designed to answer the following questions:

1. What are its characteristics of absorption, metabolism and excretion in man?

2. Are they modified by formulation, disease, prolonged administration or other drug treatment?

3. Does the drug possess in man the pharmacological properties shown in animal studies?

4. What is its optimum dose and frequency of administration?

5. What is its therapeutic ratio, that is, the ratio between the expected therapeutic dose and that producing unacceptable adverse effects? What are its specific *dose-dependent* adverse effects, and what is the incidence of *dose-independent* effects?

6. What is its mechanism of action?

This type of trial involves depth studies in relatively few subjects and it is usual for the first of these subjects to be normal volunteers in order for the normal characteristics of the drug to be assessed and compared with those which are modified by disease. This is a relatively new branch of medical science and novel methodology for careful measurement of the effects of drugs in man and for determining their mechanism of action is being developed.

It is important that those taking part in a pilot trial of this type, both normal subjects and patients, should be true volunteers without any coercion. Their informed consent should be obtained after careful explanation of the purpose of the investigation, the procedures to be used, and the risks involved. Most institutions in which such research is carried out have set up ethics committees composed of scientific and lay members who review proposed protocols and must give approval before studies may begin. Studies of new drugs in children and in patients with psychiatric conditions require special consideration outside the scope of this book.

Controlled trials

The pilot trial is 'open' in the sense that the investigator and subject are aware of the nature of the drug administered and of the effects it is likely to produce. If the evidence obtained in this trial is suggestive of a therapeutic effect of the new drug, the following questions must be asked:

(a) Has the compound significant therapeutic effects when compared with an identical placebo preparation?

(b) Is the new treatment as good as, or superior to, the best treatment at present available?

An answer to the first question will tell if the drug is really active therapeutically when the bias of the investigator or subject has been excluded. Even if it is active it would not be reasonable to market it commercially if it is inferior to other treatment already available, and this is the reason for the second question. A controlled clinical trial is designed to answer these questions, and usually includes four safeguards against bias: (1) double blind technique, (2) randomization of treatments, (3) matching of patients, (4) well-defined protocol.

Double blind technique

This ensures that neither the investigator nor the subject are aware of the treatment administered. Each treatment, that is the new drug, the standard drug with which it is to be compared and an inactive placebo, are prepared in such a way that they appear identical. It is important to ensure that the formulation of the standard drug, which is usually a compound in current use, provides the same 'biological availability' as the proprietary preparation. If not, then another error might be introduced, loading the result unfairly in favour of or against the new drug. Biological availability (or bioavailability) in this context means the facility with which a drug can be absorbed from the gastrointestinal tract (or its site of injection if administered parenterally). This may be influenced markedly by the excipient substances, or fillers, present in the tablet or capsule to provide bulk (p. 10), even though they may lack significant pharmacological activity and may not appear to influence the cruder tests of tablet disintegration and dissolution. Another use of the term bioavailability is in the comparison of the blood levels of a drug reached after intravenous administration with those reached after administration of the same dose by some other route (see p. 12). In many situations, it is not ethical to compare a new preparation with a placebo, e.g. in the treatment of a cardiac dysrhythmia or tonic-clonic seizures. Here, comparison with an appropriate active treatment prepared in a matching formulation is appropriate.

Randomization of treatments

Controlled trials may be divided into (a) within-subjects trials in which all patients receive each treatment and their responses to each are compared and (b) between-subjects trials where one patient receives only one treatment, the mean responses of each group of patients being compared. The type of trial used depends primarily on the nature of the condition which is being treated. In a chronic condition such as hypertension or rheumatoid arthritis a within-subjects study may be reasonable because a patient may be expected to return to a clinical base line when treatment is discontinued. In conditions which are self-limiting or cyclical in nature, however, such as the common cold or psychiatric states such as anxiety or depression, this assumption cannot be made and so it is not reasonable to compare treatments in the same patient. The advantage of a within-subjects trial is that it usually requires fewer subjects to reach a decision. Randomization of treatments is necessary for two reasons: (a) it avoids observer bias, and (b) it minimizes 'carry-over' effects in within-subjects trials. The administration of one drug may influence the action of subsequent treatments in a variety of ways and so disguise their true effects.

Matching of patients

Among the factors which influence a patient's response to drugs are age, sex, duration and severity of the condition which is being treated. In order to obtain a valid comparison of the activities of various preparations, therefore, and where a between-subjects comparison is necessary, it is desirable to match patients between treatment groups for these various factors. This may prove difficult if the condition is relatively uncommon or tends to occur in one sex more than the other or in one particular age group. A patient's weight may also be an important determining factor in response to a drug. In animal experiments it is usual to administer a drug on the basis of body weight but in therapeutic practice in man this is seldom done except where toxicity is high and dose-related. In fixed-dose studies blood and tissue levels of a drug tend to be higher in lighter subjects, which may produce differences in therapeutic response and toxicity. It is wise, therefore, to match patients for weight whenever possible, or to relate the dose given to their weight.

Well-defined protocol

Before commencing a clinical trial, it is important to define carefully, in writing, the methods to be used in measurement of the appropriate parameters, the details of times of drug administration and various recordings, and the criteria which are considered necessary for inclusion of a subject in the trial and for the assessment of his response to treatment. Once such a protocol has been carefully prepared it should be adhered to throughout the trial.

Statistical analysis

The final stage of a clinical trial is the statistical analysis of the results obtained. Although relatively simple tests such as Chi-squared, Student's t and ranking methods may be sufficient where large and obvious differences appear between treatments, more sophisticated methods are available which may show significant differences which are not so readily apparent. Multi-variate techniques of analysis of variance, covariance and dispersion are particularly valuable, for they minimize differences in results due to other factors (such as between-subjects and between-times variations) so that the between-treatment differences are emphasized. These methods are complicated, however, particularly when several different factors are being assessed, and expert help and computer facilities are almost always required.

Although it is desirable to assess the effects of a drug in terms of units of measurement, for example heart rate, blood pressure, body weight or urine volume, there are many types of trial where this is not possible, particularly in investigation of drugs in psychiatry. This may depend on the global judgement of the investigator, as for example, whether a patient is improved or deteriorating. There may also be important ethical reasons for discontinuing a trial as soon as a statistically significant result is obtained, for example in the treatment of malignant conditions. In such circumstances the *sequential trial* may be appropriate. This involves making preferences for one form of treatment against another, either within-patients or between matched patients, and plotting them on a graph prepared from special tables, when the statistical requirements for significance have been decided. When a line of significance is crossed, either for one drug against another, or of no difference between treatments, then the trial can be discontinued. Figure 1

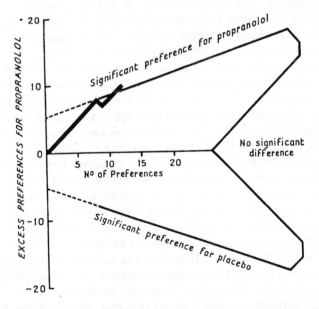

Fig. 1 Chart of sequential study for investigator's preferences in a trial of propranolol *v.* placebo in anxiety state. ($\theta = 0.8$, $2a = 0.8$, $2a = 0.05$, and $\beta = 0.05$.) (Reproduced from K. L. Granville-Grossman & P. Turner (1966). *Lancet* i, 788–790, by kind permission of the editor.)

shows such a sequential graph in which propranolol was shown to be significantly superior to placebo in anxious patients after only fifteen preferences had been made, in a double-blind randomized within-patient (cross-over) trial. For most types of investigation of this kind, a probability figure of 5 per cent is usually taken as being significant, so that the chances of obtaining a positive result when in fact it does not really exist are less than 5 per cent, while on the other hand the chances of not obtaining a positive result when one really exists are also less than 5 per cent.

Statistical techniques are complex, and wrong conclusions may be reached if an inappropriate one is chosen for a particular problem. For this reason it is wise to include a statistician in the team when planning and carrying out a clinical trial.

Monitored release and post-marketing surveillance

Identification of the syndrome of adverse reactions associated with the long-term use of practolol (p. 51) emphasised the importance of close surveillance of large numbers of patients receiving new drugs over a period of many years. Recognition of the practolol syndrome was delayed because it had not previously been associated with other drugs, nor had it been produced in animal models. This demonstrates the necessity to record carefully all clinical events, and the patients' responses to life events such as other illness, pregnancy and bereavement, in sufficient numbers of patients to detect relatively uncommon reactions, over a period of time sufficient to detect long-term adverse effects in the patients or in their offspring. An example of the importance of the latter is the increased incidence of vaginal carcinoma in adolescent daughters of women given stilboestrol early in pregnancy (p. 189).

Several schemes have been proposed to permit identification of patients prescribed a new drug, and regular notification of their clinical progress to central monitoring agencies. Some depend on the assistance of dispensing pharmacists in recording the names of patients prescribed the particular drug. Others seek to exploit the prescription pricing agencies employed in health and welfare services such as the National Health Service in Britain to identify the prescriptions for the drugs under surveillance. Yet others place the responsibility for identifying the patient population on the pharmaceutical company which markets the drug. Every scheme, however, depends for its ultimate success on careful clinical scrutiny of the patient by the prescribing doctor, the meticulous recording of his observations in the patients' documents, and a high index of suspicion that any unexpected clinical event may be associated with a drug's administration.

2

Factors influencing the action of drugs

If a fixed dose of a drug is prescribed for a number of patients with a particular disease (e.g. 300 mg of phenytoin daily in patients with epilepsy) most will show some degree of therapeutic response. A few, however, will not be obviously improved, while the occasional patient may gradually develop signs of drug intoxication. Although the severity of the disease itself may vary from one patient to another, this difference in response is largely accounted for by variations in the metabolic handling of the drug.

If the serum level of phenytoin is measured in these patients a tenfold difference may be found at the two extremes. It would not be surprising, therefore, if some patients were undertreated while others were intoxicated. A number of factors are responsible for this phenomenon, apart from failure to take the prescribed dose of the drug (and this is one of the chief reasons for therapeutic failure in outpatients). The rate and extent of absorption of the drug, its distribution in the various body compartments, tissue and plasma-protein binding, and the rate of metabolism and excretion of the drug all influence the steady-state level of the drug at the site where it is required. Study of these aspects of pharmacology (called pharmacokinetics) has become increasingly important in recent years, and leads to a more precise regulation of drug therapy.

Formulation of drugs into medicines
Many doctors do not realize that when they prescribe a *drug* the patient actually receives a *medicine*. The active substance represents only a small proportion of the total weight of an oral solid dosage form such as a tablet or capsule. Similarly, the form of a drug for injection requires solution or suspension in a fluid vehicle of varying complexity. The other constituents of dosage forms are not necessarily 'inert', however, but may play an important part in facilitating or hindering a drug's absorption. Furthermore, appropriate manipulation of these materials may permit development of sophisticated delivery systems for delayed or position-release of the

drug. The following are some of the more important factors which are involved in the production of tablets and capsules, which may influence a drug's absorption.

1. Diluents such as lactose or calcium sulphate are used to increase bulk. The importance of these particular diluents in determining the rate of absorption of phenytoin was demonstrated by an outbreak of phenytoin intoxication in Australia when the formulation was changed from one to the other.

2. Granulating and binding agents, such as tragacanth or syrup are used to assist aggregation of the powder into granules, in order to permit compression into tablets. Bentonite is a naturally occurring mineral consisting chiefly of hydrated aluminium silicate, which is employed pharmaceutically as a binder. It has been shown to adsorb rifampicin rapidly and strongly, and so can significantly decrease the absorption of rifampicin if given simultaneously, for example, in PAS granules in which it has been used to aid granulation.

3. Lubricants, such as talc, prevent granule adherence to the tablet punches.

4. Disintegrating agents are incorporated to produce rapid tablet disintegration in the gastrointestinal tract. They include substances such as starch which swell on contact with moisture, substances such as cocoa butter which melt at body temperature, and others such as a mixture of sodium bicarbonate and tartaric acid which effervesce on contact with moisture.

5. Coating materials such as sugar may be used to prevent disintegration before the tablet reaches the stomach or intestine, as well as for cosmetic and identification purposes.

6. Capsules have a gelatin envelope and do not involve granulating excipients. It is a common misapprehension that drugs are released more rapidly from capsule than from tablets; this is not necessarily so.

7. Special formulations employ complex pharmaceutical manoeuvres to control disintegration and dissolution rates, so regulating the rate of a drug's absorption. This has lead to the development of sustained release and of position release formulations.

8. As well as the foregoing non-drug factors, different manufacturing processes may result in the production of different physical forms of the active drug, and this may influence its rates of dissolution and absorption. The absorption rates of griseofulvin and digoxin, among others, have been shown to be related to particle size.

These matters are relevant to the question of whether generic or brand names should be used in prescribing. The generic or 'approved' name does not necessarily determine the formulation which the patient will receive. Use of the brand name should determine not only the physical form of the drug, but also the excipients and method of manufacture which may influence absorption. Where differences in biological availability of a drug have been shown to be important in patient care, it may be wise to use the proprietary brand name rather than is generic name in prescribing.

Patient compliance

This describes the extent to which a patient carries out the wishes of his prescribing doctor in taking his medication, and is an important determinant of therapeutic outcome of treatment. It is influenced by the dosage form, frequency of administration, number of drugs prescribed and adverse drug effects, as well as by the patient's age and ability to comprehend instructions.

Absorption of drugs

An orally administered drug must pass through the bowel wall in order to enter the bloodstream. This barrier is a complex lipid membrane composed of the walls of the cells lining the bowel. Substances, whether food or drugs, can pass through this membrane in one of four ways:

(a) Passive diffusion, by which the substance passes through the membrane in solution; diffusion is proportional to the concentration difference across the membrane and the lipid solubility of the drug.

(b) Active transport, by which substances (e.g. amino acids) are carried across the membrane by an energy-consuming mechanism, usually against a concentration gradient; some drugs, because of their resemblance to naturally-occurring substances, utilize existing transport systems (e.g. α -methyl dopa).

(c) Filtration through pores, which is limited to molecules of small size (e.g. urea).

(d) Pinocytosis, by which small particles are engulfed by cells of the bowel wall.

Of these four mechanisms the first, passive diffusion, is by far the most important for drug absorption. Considering, then, this mechanism in particular, there are a number of factors which will influence absorption:

1. The chemical nature of the drug. Polypeptides (e.g. insulin)

are broken down by intestinal enzymes, while benzylpenicillin is destroyed by gastric acid. Large, lipid-insoluble molecules for which no active system exists are poorly absorbed (e.g. mersalyl).

2. Formulation (see p. 9).

3. pH. Most commonly-used drugs are either weak acids or weak bases, and these exist in two forms in solution, as undissociated molecules and as ions. The equilibrium between these two forms is determined by (a) the pK value of the drug and (b) the pH of the surrounding medium. At a pH equal to the pK the drug is 50 per cent ionized. At a low pH (i.e. in the stomach) a weakly acidic drug will be mainly in its undissociated form, whereas a weakly basic drug will be largely ionized. In a more alkaline medium (i.e. in the small bowel) the reverse applies. As only the undissociated molecules are appreciably lipid-soluble an acid medium favours the absorption of weakly acidic drugs, while weak bases are better absorbed from the small intestine. A few drugs (e.g. streptomycin and hexamethonium) are strongly basic and their pK values greatly exceed the highest pH reached in the intestine. As these drugs remain ionized throughout the alimentary tract they are very poorly absorbed. Although these general rules explain the behaviour of most drugs, there are some which do not obey these principles for a variety of reasons. For example, sulphaguanidine is very poorly absorbed, not because it remains ionized in the gut, but because its undissociated form is poorly lipid-soluble. Dicoumarol, although highly lipid-soluble, is poorly absorbed because it is relatively insoluble in the alimentary fluid.

4. Gut motility. Most drugs are absorbed from the upper part of the small bowel, and alterations in gut motility can markedly influence drug absorption (see p. 161).

5. Food. Dilution of the drug by food and drink, and the delay in gastric emptying produced by a meal, lead to a slowing of absorption of most drugs. Unless a drug is irritant to the stomach, it should be taken on an empty stomach. There are, however, some exceptions, e.g. griseofulvin is better absorbed after a fatty meal.

6. Liver and bowel wall enzymes. Unless a drug is absorbed directly into the systemic circulation, as from sublingual or rectal administration, it has to pass through the liver in the portal circulation. Some drugs, e.g. propranolol, lignocaine, chlormethiazole, oestrogens are extensively metabolized as they pass through the liver—the so-called 'first-pass effect'. Induction of first-pass metabolism can reduce the amount of drug available systemically.

All these factors influence the 'biological availability' of a drug, that is, the facility with which it is absorbed into the bloodstream.

Distribution and protein binding

As a general rule, those drugs which are readily absorbed from the gastrointestinal tract are freely and rapidly distributed throughout the body water compartments. Diazepam is highly lipid-soluble and is freely absorbed from stomach or rectum. When injected intravenously it passes rapidly through lipid barriers into the brain to terminate status epilepticus. It follows that centrally-acting drugs, because they have to enter the brain through a lipid membrane, are usually readily absorbed from the gastrointestinal tract. The same drugs, however, can easily gain access to the foetal circulation, and for this reason centrally-acting drugs are the chief offenders in causing foetal abnormalities (e.g. phocomelia caused by thalidomide).

Many drugs are loosely bound to plasma and tissue proteins, and the extent of this binding will affect the kinetics of the drug in question. For a drug showing no appreciable binding the tissues act as little more than a water compartment in which the drug is dissolved. Extensive plasma and tissue protein binding will increase the quantity of the drug which has to be absorbed before effective therapeutic levels of unbound drug are reached at the site of action. A period of many days may be required for equilibration between the body fluids and tissues. A drug which is extensively bound to tissues is said to have a large 'apparent volume of distribution' (V_d). This is a theoretical volume of fluid which would be required to contain the total body content of drug at a concentration equal to the plasma concentration. Nortriptyline is an example of a drug which is extensively tissue bound; its V_d is around 20 litres/kg. Warfarin, on the other hand, has a V_d of only $0\cdot1$ litres/kg.

Elimination by metabolism and excretion may be delayed when tissue binding is extensive because V_d is one determinant of the plasma half life ($t\frac{1}{2}$). The greater the quantity of drug requiring elimination, the longer the time to eliminate it completely. The rate of metabolism, as well as the pharmacological effect of a drug, is determined by the concentration of unbound drug in the plasma. However, there are exceptions. When the rate limiting step in metabolism is the delivery of drug to the liver, as it is for propranolol, plasma protein binding may actually enhance elimination. The former situation is known as 'restrictive' elimination, while the latter is called 'non-restrictive'.

Changes in the concentration of plasma proteins will reduce the amount of drug bound, and consequently the total plasma concentration (free plus bound) will be lower than expected for a given pharmacological effect. Renal disease can reduce the binding capacity of albumin; the reason for this is uncertain but a change in configuration of the molecule is possible. Drugs can compete for plasma protein binding sites and this may lead to a transient increase in effect for drugs with a small V_d. Competition for tissue binding sites has been little studied.

Serum levels

When a drug has been absorbed from the alimentary tract, and distribution to the tissues has taken place, its concentration in the plasma falls along an exponential time course. A semi-logarithmic plot of serum concentration against time will produce a straight line relationship, from which can be obtained the half-life of the drug, i.e. the time taken for the serum concentration to halve. The duration of this half-life is determined by the rate of elimination of the drug by metabolism or excretion, and by V_d (see above). When a drug is injected intravenously, the serum concentration decays initially in a complex manner, being dependent first of all on distribution to the various body compartments. Subsequently, however, an exponential fall resembling that after an oral dose occurs. The half-life of a drug must be taken into account in determining the frequency of dosage. Salbutamol has a short half-life and produces a much steadier therapeutic action if given in at least three divided doses daily. Digoxin, however, has a long half-life and giving the drug as a single daily dose is adequate to maintain a steady response. Drugs with a long half-life will be cumulative with repeated and frequent dosage, and patients receiving drugs like digoxin, guanethidine or phenytoin should be examined frequently for signs of overdosage. Measurements of serum concentrations are made routinely with only few drugs at present, although there is a good case for regular estimations with many drugs, particularly anticonvulsant and antidysrhythmic drugs, theophylline, lithium and the aminoglycosides, and more facilities for this will undoubtedly become available in the future. In some cases, measuring the response to a drug provides an easy method of monitoring its action (e.g. prothrombin time with anticoagulants).

Metabolism

Most drugs administered to man are metabolized by liver enzymes, although, in addition, some are destroyed by enzymes in the plasma or other tissues (e.g. procaine is destroyed by pseudocholinesterase in the serum). Metabolism in the liver occurs particularly with those drugs which are lipid soluble and can therefore readily enter the liver cells. At first sight it seems surprising that the liver has enzyme systems ready and waiting to metabolize any foreign substance in the form of a drug. However, the pathways for breakdown of both intrinsic and extrinsic substances are relatively stereotyped, and each is specific for certain chemical groups which can occur on a wide variety of substances. The object of these processes is to produce derivatives of increasing polarity which are less lipid-soluble and can be excreted by the kidney (see below).

Drugs possessing a hydroxyl, carboxyl or amino group are usually conjugated to form a glucuronide, an ethereal sulphate or a glycine or acetyl derivative. Drugs lacking one of those groups are usually oxidized, dealkylated, deaminated or hydroxylated, and subsequent conjugation often occurs. Occasionally, a metabolite of a drug is pharmacologically active, and may account largely for the therapeutic action of the drug (e.g. primidone is metabolized to phenobarbitone, which is largely responsible for the anticonvulsant activity of the parent drug). Because enzymes are used in common by many different intrinsic and extrinsic substances, it is not surprising that interaction between these compounds can occur at this level (liver enzyme induction and inhibition are discussed in Chapter 3). Furthermore, impaired hepatic function must be taken into consideration before administration of any drug which depends on the liver for its degradation. In general, however, liver disease has to be severe before a clinically important slowing of drug metabolism occurs.

Excretion

Most drugs are eventually excreted in the urine, either as the parent substance or as metabolites. Drugs which are well absorbed from the alimentary tract (i.e. lipid-soluble drugs) appear in the glomerular filtrate, but readily pass back into the bloodstream by passive diffusion at the proximal tubule. As has been mentioned above, many of these drugs are converted by the liver into more polar, lipid-insoluble metabolites. These metabolites, and other drugs which are highly polar (e.g. hexamethonium), do not pass very readily into the glomerular filtrate, but once they are there they have difficulty in diffusing back at the proximal tubule. Thus, these substances are usually eliminated entirely by renal excretion. In addition to passive diffusion, many acidic and basic drugs are actively secreted by the renal tubules. The secretion of weakly acidic substances can be inhibited by probenecid, and this substance has been used to prolong the half-life of penicillin in order to reach higher tissue concentrations without increasing the dose of the antibiotic.

Because tubular reabsorption by passive diffusion limits the excretion of many lipid soluble drugs, changes in tubular pH can affect the elimination of these compounds by altering the ratio of ionized to unionized form. Normally the urine is slightly acid and favours the excretion of weakly basic drugs (e.g. amphetamine. Further acidification of the urine by giving ammonium chloride orally demonstrably shortens the action of these drugs, while oral sodium bicarbonate will prolong their effects. The reverse applies for weakly acidic drugs, and this is the reason why an alkaline diuresis has been used in accelerating the elimination of phenobarbitone, or aspirin in patients who have taken an overdose. The effect, however, appears to be small with most of these drugs, and is in itself a hazardous procedure.

As the kidney is so important in drug excretion, care must be exercised in patients with impaired renal function. An elderly patient with congestive cardiac failure and a raised blood urea is likely to develop digitalis intoxication if digoxin is prescribed in full dosage. It is necessary to measure repeatedly the serum level of certain drugs (e.g. gentamicin) when they are given to patients in renal failure.

Some drugs (e.g. novobiocin, erythromycin, carbenoxolone) are secreted in the bile and reabsorbed. This 'entero-hepatic' circulation can lead to very high blood levels with repeated dosage. The action of phenolphthalein is prolonged by this mechanism.

Dosage interval

With repeated dosing, for practical purposes it takes five half-lives before a steady-state serum level is reached. To give an example, digoxin has a $t^{1/2}$ of 36 hours on average, and therefore at least one week of therapy is required before a steady effect is obtained. If an immediate effect is necessary, a loading dose can be given at the outset. The size of the load is determined mainly by body weight, whereas the subsequent maintenance doses are judged by the elimination rate, which in the case of digoxin will be proportional to the creatinine clearance. Both the loading and maintenance doses can be estimated with the use of nomograms. Loading doses are necessary only with a few drugs, and then only in certain situations, e.g. oral anticoagulants, aminoglycosides in severe systemic infections, and phenytoin in status epilepticus.

The degree to which a drug accumulates on repeated dosing depends upon its plasma $t^{1/2}$. Penicillin, for example, has a $t^{1/2}$ of only 30 minutes and even with 4-hourly administration it will accumulate little because for practical purposes the antibiotic is practically eliminated in less than the dose interval. At the other extreme is a drug like phenobarbitone, which has a $t^1/_2$ of about four days in adults. Even with once daily administration, much of the previous dose is still present in the body when subsequent doses are given, and therefore accumulation is marked. Steady-state will be reached only after about three weeks of continuous therapy.

3

Adverse effects of drugs

Any substance which possesses useful therapeutic effects may also produce unwanted, toxic, or adverse effects in certain individuals and if taken in sufficient quantities. The incidence of adverse drug effects in the population is unknown because of difficulties of monitoring them, but it is certainly not small and much morbidity and discomfort is produced by drug treatment. Studies of the incidence of fatal drug reactions in hospital have suggested that about 0·5 per cent of patients who die in hospital do so as a result of their treatment rather than the condition for which they were admitted.

Although there are many different ways of classifying adverse drug effects, the simplest is probably to divide them into those which are (a) dose-independent and (b) dose-dependent. All drugs produce both types of effect to a varying degree.

DOSE-INDEPENDENT EFFECTS

These occur in only a small proportion of patients, and tend to be limited to certain well-defined manifestations. The most common are *hypersensitivity reactions* due to release of histamine or histamine-like substances causing rashes, oedema or more serious effects such as bronchospasm, peripheral vasodilation and cardiovascular collapse, the *anaphylactic reaction*. This reaction is due to previous sensitization of the patient to the drug or to some other substance which possesses cross-antigenicity with it. For example, exposure to one form of penicillin usually produces a state of hypersensitivity to other penicillin derivatives. Another form of dose-independent adverse drug reaction is the production of blood dyscrasias, the most important of which are aplastic anaemia, agranulocytosis, thrombocytopenia and haemolytic anaemia. Chloramphenicol is a very effective antiobiotic but about one person in every 20 000 develops a fatal aplastic anaemia which is unrelated to the dose administered. Unfortunately, no satisfactory test exists at present which can safely be carried out on patients to determine if they will react in one of these ways to a particular drug.

DOSE-DEPENDENT EFFECTS

These occur in all patients given the drug if it is administered in sufficiently large doses, which may vary considerably from patient to patient. Whereas the dose-independent effects are non-specific, of the types described above, dose-dependent effects tend to be specific for the drug. Some are predictable, being exaggerated therapeutic actions, for example the depression of cardiac contractility by quinidine. Others may be unrelated to their therapeutic effects, for example the ototoxicity produced by streptomycin. Dose-dependent effects are influenced by several factors:

1. Age

Some drugs produce unexpected adverse effects at the extremes of life.

(a) Drugs given in the first three months of pregnancy, during the period of organogenesis, may cause congenital abnormalities, and are said to be *teratogenic*. Very few drugs have been proven to possess teratogenic activity, the most well-known being thalidomide. Others are antineoplastic drugs (such as aminopterin, methotrexate, 6-mercaptopurine and cyclophosphamide) which produce a variety of malformations or lead to abortion, and cortisone which may produce cleft palate. The use of anticonvulsant drugs in major epilepsy is associated with an increase in the incidence of congenital abnormalities, particularly hare lip and cleft palate. Sex hormones, both androgens and oestrogens may cause virilizing effects in female foetuses if given to the mother in early pregnancy. Lysergic acid diethylamide may produce chromosomal damage in the foetus, and it is suspected that this may lead to congenital defects. The type of congenital abnormality produced by teratogenic agents depends primarily on the time of administration in terms of the development stages of the embryo. For example, in the human embryo, the critical teratogenic period for the nervous system is between days 15 and 25, for the eye 24 to 40, for the heart 20 to 40 and for the legs 24 to 36.

(b) Drugs given after the period of organogenesis may affect the growth or function of normally-formed foetal tissues or organs.

Among the more important are:

Antibacterial drugs. Tetracyclines may become concentrated in foetal bones to impair growth and in teeth to produce discolouration and increased susceptibility to caries. Streptomycin and gentamicin may damage the foetal labyrinth and auditory nerve. Long-acting sulphonamides and novobiocin, which are extensively bound to plasma proteins, may compete successfully with bilirubin for binding sites, displacing it and leading to severe jaundice or kernicterus.

Antithyroid drugs. Maternal ingestion of antithyroid drugs and iodides may produce foetal or neonatal hypothyroidism and goitre.

Anticoagulants. The foetus appears to be very sensitive to the oral anticoagulants of the coumarin and indandione groups, and foetal or neonatal haemorrhage may occur, even though the maternal prothrombin time is within the safe range.

Oral hypoglycaemic drugs. Sulphonylurea drugs may produce foetal hypoglycaemia and intrauterine death.

Cardiovascular drugs. Sympathomimetic drugs may adversely affect the foetus. Beta-receptor stimulants such as isoprenaline may produce foetal tachycardia and alpha-receptor agonists may cause foetal anoxia indirectly due to uterine vasoconstriction. Beta-receptor blocking drugs such as propranolol can produce foetal bradycardia. Ganglion blocking drugs may produce hypotension and paralytic ileus in the neonate, and reserpine given a few days before delivery can cause bradycardia and nasal stuffiness which can lead to respiratory distress.

Labour. Nearly all the analgesics, sedatives, hypnotics and anaesthetics, both general and local, administered to a mother during labour, can adversely affect the neonate.

(c) Neonate, infants and children

Drug metabolizing enzymes may be deficient for at least a month after birth, and this is particularly marked in the premature neonate. Neonates are said to have problems in metabolizing effectively vitamin K analogues, sulphonamides, barbiturates, morphine and curare. One of the most dramatic examples is the production by chloramphenicol of the 'grey baby syndrome' in premature infants. This is a form of circulatory collapse and muscular hypotonia, and appears to be due to a combination of defective conjugation of chloramphenicol in the liver, and accumulation of unconjugated drug because of immature renal excretion. There is considerable evidence that foetal metabolizing activity can be induced (see p. 23) in the newborn babies of mothers treated during pregnancy with, for example, anticonvulsants such as phenytoin.

Once the liver enzymes have matured in the neonate, the rate of drug metabolism becomes greater than in the adult and this persists throughout childhood, although gradually diminishing until adult stature is reached at adolescence. This may be due, at least in part, to the fact that the ratio of liver weight to body weight in children may be 30–50 per cent greater than in adults.

Although the foetal kidney is able to excrete sodium and concentrate urea from as early as 14 weeks gestation, newborn infants have a relatively lower glomerular filtration rate and renal plasma flow than adults. The maintenance doses of all drugs eliminated from the body by renal excretion of the active compound should, therefore, be very low during the first few days of life and low during the next few weeks while renal function is maturing.

Drugs secreted into breast milk may be absorbed by the infant during breast feeding. Factors influencing their concentration in milk include plasma protein binding, pKa and partition coefficient.

(d) Old age

Many groups of drugs produce more adverse effects in elderly patients. Central depressant compounds such as sedatives, tranquillizers and hypnotics are more liable to produce confusional states. This is due, in part, to reduced hepatic extraction and metabolism of drugs which has been demonstrated with increasing age, but also to age-related changes in the sensitivity of the central nervous system to the effects of these compounds.

Glomerular filtration rate falls with age, even in apparently healthy subjects, and this can lead to cumulation of drugs which are principally excreted unchanged by the kidney. This probably is the main cause for the increased sensitivity to the action of digitalis seen in elderly patients, and maintenance doses for the young or middle-aged patient often produce marked toxicity in the elderly.

Another important factor to be considered is that increasing age is associated with changes in body composition as well as to a general tendency to a decrease in body weight, and these factors may influence the distribution and tissue levels of administered drugs.

(e) Compliance (see p. 11).

2 Enzyme abnormalities
These are either inherited or acquired.

(a) Inherited
An increasing number of adverse drug reactions are being shown to be due to hereditary enzymatic variations, and some of these are summarized in Table 1.

Among other adverse reactions of drugs which may depend on inherited enzyme abnormalities are the exacerbation of acute intermittent porphyria by barbiturates and the rare occurrence of familial resistance to coumarin anticoagulants.

Table 1

Enzyme deficient	Geographical features	Drugs involved	Adverse effects
Cholinesterase (Serum or pseudocholinesterase)	World-wide	Succinylcholine	Neuromuscular blockade and apnoea
Liver N-acetyltransferase	World-wide	Isoniazid Procainamide Phenelzine Hydralazine	Polyneuritis Systemic lupus erythematosus
Glucose-6-phosphate dehydrogenase	Mediterranean and Negro races, Sephardic Jews	Primaquine Sulphonamides Nitrofurantoin Quinine Chloramphenicol Fava beans	Haemolysis
Erythrocye diaphorase (methaemoglobin reductase)	World-wide	Sulphonamides Nitrites	Methaemoglobinaemia

(b) Acquired

Enzyme inhibition. The most important example of adverse reactions due to enzyme inhibition is associated with the administration of the monoamine oxidase inhibitors (MAOI). These are a heterogeneous group of drugs which have in common the ability to block the activity of monoamine oxidase. This is a widely distributed enzyme responsible for the intracellular degradation of adrenaline, noradrenaline and dopamine, and also of 5-hydroxy-tryptamine and other monoamines. As a result, particular care must be exercised when the following are taken by patients receiving MAOIs.

(i) Sympathomimetic amines. Indirectly acting amines act by releasing noradrenaline from adrenergic nerve terminals. After MAO inhibition their peripheral and central effects are potentiated, probably because there are increased stores of noradrenaline to be released, and their own biotransformation is reduced. Many easily obtainable proprietary remedies for upper respiratory tract infections contain these amines, and patients taking MAOIs must be advised to be cautious in their use. The clinical results of such interactions include central stimulation, anxiety, restlessness, headache, hypertension, chest pain and cardiac dysrhythmias.

(ii) Certain foodstuffs. Foods which contain indirectly-acting amines may produce hypertensive reactions in patients taking MAOIs. Among these are broad beans containing DOPA, and cheeses, wines, meat and yeast products and chicken liver which all contain tyramine.

(iii) Dibenzazepine drugs. This group of antidepressant drugs, including imipramine, nortriptyline and amitriptyline, are thought to act by inhibiting the uptake of noradrenaline into adrenergic nerve terminals, so increasing its activity at the receptor site. It would be expected on theoretical grounds, therefore, that MAOIs might potentiate their effects, and this has been demonstrated in animal experiments. There have also been reports of serious reactions including agitation, hyperpyrexia, convulsions and circulatory collapse in patients treated with a combination of both groups of drugs.

(iv) Antihypertensive drugs. Drugs such as reserpine, guanethidine and bethanidine which deplete peripheral stores of noradrenaline may, in the absence of MAO activity, release increased amounts of noradrenaline on to receptor sites, producing hypertension and its acute complications.

(v) Pethidine. If patients receiving MAOIs are given pethidine in normal therapeutic doses there may be severe toxic reactions including excitement and hyperthermia. Animal experiments suggest that these effects are associated with raised levels of cerebral 5-hydroxytryptamine rather than noradrenaline.

Enzyme induction. The magnitude and duration of action of many drugs as well as endogenously produced substances are dependent on the rate of their biotransformation by the drug metabolizing enzymes of the liver. The activity of these enzymes may be increased by treatment with a large number of commonly used substances including insecticides and pesticides. This is accompanied in animals by increased liver weight and increased production of microsomal protein. Reactions which may be associated with this phenomenon are shown in Table 2.

Table 2

Chief drugs causing enzyme induction	Drugs whose metabolism is affected	Result
Barbiturates, particularly long-acting	Oral anticoagulants	Reduced and unpredictable anticoagulant effect
Glutethimide	Corticosteriods	Reduced effect in asthma
MANDRAX	Sex hormones (e.g. the 'pill')	Contraceptive failure
Phenytoin		
Primidone	Vitamin D	Osteomalacia or rickets
Carbamazepine	Tricyclic antidepressants	Reduced psychotropic effect
Rifampicin	Phenothiazines	
	Antipyrine (phenazone)	Shortened half-life (used as index of liver enzyme induction)

3. Protein binding displacement

A proportion of most drugs in the plasma is bound to protein. Certain groups of drugs appear to share a limited number of common binding sites and one can compete with and displace another. Sometimes an increase in the effect of the drug occurs because the free concentration may be significantly increased, but the extent of this is determined by the apparent volume of distribution of the drug. When the latter is large the quantity of drug displaced from plasma proteins is negligible in comparison and the free concentration of drug increases little (e.g. phenytoin displaced by sodium valproate). When the volume of distribution is small (e.g. warfarin) the increase may produce measurable effects although these are seldom important. However, the increase is only transient because the rise in free concentration causes an increase in metabolism which restores the original free concentration. The free *fraction* (i.e. the ratio of free to bound drug) will remain increased when a new equilibrium has been reached, but the *total* serum concentration will be lower than before the interaction occurred, and this may have implications for drugs that are monitored on a routine basis for clinical purposes (e.g. phenytoin).

Phenylbutazone, aspirin and sulphonamides can displace warfarin, and sometimes an increase in anticoagulation may occur, but this may partly be explained by a simultaneous inhibition of metabolism. Tolbutamide, for instance, is known to have both effects.

4. Liver disease

Liver disease is important in drug toxicity in two ways:

(a) Certain drugs may precipitate hepatic encephalopathy in patients with poor liver function. Chief among these are potassium-losing diuretics such as the thiazides and frusemide, narcotic analgesics and drugs which depress the central nervous system.

(b) The action of drugs whose main route of metabolism and inactivation is in the liver may be increased in degree and duration. These include corticosteroids, narcotic analgesics, several barbiturates and the phenothiazine drugs. The action of oral anticoagulants, too, may be affected in this way, but here there is the added potentiating factor of reduced prothrombin synthesis in liver disease which leads to further reduction of prothrombin activity. Hypoalbuminaemia may also contribute by increasing the level of unbound drug in the plasma. Portal-systemic shunting in hepatic cirrhosis can increase the plasma levels of some drugs (e.g. propranolol) which normally have an extensive first-pass metabolism.

In general, however, the impairment of drug metabolism in liver disease is unpredictable and is usually less clinically important than the other consequences of liver failure.

Drug induced jaundice

Jaundice due to drugs may, like other adverse effects, be dose-dependent or dose-independent in origin. It may also, like other forms of jaundice due to liver dysfunction, be hepatocellular or cholestatic in type. Some examples of each are given in Table 3.

Table 3 Drug-induced liver disease

	Hepatocellular	Cholestatic
Dose-dependent	Cytostatic drugs Paracetamol Phenylbutazone	Methyl testosterone
Dose-independent	Monoamine oxidase inhibitors Halothane	Chlorpropamide Phenothiazines Phenindione Erythromycin estolate

5. Renal disease

Drugs which are eliminated partly or entirely in the urine will accumulate when renal function is impaired, increasing the likelihood of dose-related adverse effects. For drugs which have a narrow therapeutic ratio and are eliminated entirely by the kidney, a major reduction in dose is required, whereas less toxic drugs may be prescribed in standard doses unless renal function is severely impaired (Table 4). Some drugs should be avoided altogether if renal function is impaired because they are nephro-toxic or because the risk of adverse effects is too great. Potassium supplements, preparations containing large amounts of sodium (e.g. p-amino salicyclic acid), and magnesium salts (e.g. magnesium trisilicate, magnesium sulphate) should be used with caution because of the danger of accumulation.

Plasma protein binding may be reduced in renal failure, leading to toxicity even though the total plasma level remains within the therapeutic range (e.g. phenytoin, tricyclic antidepressants).

6. Route of administration

The route of administration may be important in determining dose-dependent adverse reactions, a well-known example being the

Table 4 Drugs in renal disease

Drug	Adverse effect
Avoid altogether	
Tetracylines ⎫	
Cephaloridine ⎬	Nephrotoxicity
Amphotericin ⎭	
Ethacrynic acid	Deafness following IV injection
Chlorpropamide	Hypoglycaemia
Nitrofurantoin	Neurotoxicity
Dose reduction in mild renal failure	
Aminoglycoside antibiotics	Ototoxicity, nephrotoxicity
Lithium	CNS toxicity
Dose reduction in moderate	
renal failure	
Digoxin	Nausea, dysrhythmias
Cyclophosphamide	Bone marrow depression
Clofibrate	Myopathy
Penicillamine	Nephrotoxicity. Bone marrow depression
Dose reduction only in severe	
renal failure	
Penicillins	Rashes. Neurotoxicity
Co-trimoxazole ⎫	Nephrotoxicity. Bone marrow
Sulphonamides ⎬	depression
Isoniazid	Peripheral neuropathy
Tolbutamide	Hypoglycaemia

tissue necrosis produced by thiopentone when administered intra-arterially rather than intravenously. Intrathecal penicillin has caused many deaths from encephalopathy and convulsions because the doctor injecting the drug did not realize that the intrathecal dose should be only one hundredth of the intramuscular dose.

4

Mechanisms of drug interaction

It is common for patients to be treated with more than one drug at the same time, and there are several different ways in which they may interact for the patient's good or harm. The following is a general summary of some of the principal mechanisms involved.

1. Formulation incompatibility

Drugs may interact with so-called 'inert' constituents of the formulations in which they are compounded, and this may influence their biological availability (see pp. 5 and 9). This applies equally to oral and parenteral preparations.

2. Absorption

Drugs which influence the rate of gastric emptying may modify the rate of absorption of other drugs (see p. 161) Chelaton or other forms of binding of drugs within the gastrointestinal tract may reduce their absorption. Ferrous compounds and calcium, magnesium and aluminium-containing antacids chelate with tetracyclines to reduce the absorption of the latter. The anion-exchange resin cholestyramine can reduce the absorption of digoxin, thiazide diuretics, thyroxine and paracetamol.

Vasoconstrictor drugs are combined with local anaesthetic agents in some parenteral formulations to restrict their area of action at the injection site. On the other hand, a vasodilator drug may be combined with another drug to increase its rate of intramuscular absorption, as, for example, in the combination of theophylline with mersalyl.

3. Protein binding (see p. 13)

4. Enzyme induction (see p. 23)

5. Enzyme inhibition

Some drugs, such as sulthiame, may inhibit drug metabolising enzymes and so prolong the plasma half-lives of some other drugs.

Treatment with monoamine oxidase inhibitors leads to accumulation of monoamines such as adrenaline, noradrenaline, dopamine and 5-hydroxytryptamine within the central and autonomic nervous systems, and also prevents the hepatic metabolism of other exogenous monoamines such as tyramine. This is the basis of their important interactions with certain drugs and foodstuffs (see p. 22).

Organo-phosphorus anticholinesterases instilled into the conjunctival sac in the treatment of glaucoma may be absorbed sufficiently to produce resistance to neuro-muscular blockade by tubocurarine.

Enzyme inhibition is also the basis of action of many chemotherapeutic agents used in treatment of infectious and neoplastic conditions. Synergism between drugs may occur if they act on different enzyme systems within the cells of an infecting organism or in a neoplastic cell. For example, in the combination product co-trimoxazole, sulphamethoxazole inhibits the conversion of para-aminobenzoic acid to folic acid, and trimethoprim inhibits the conversion of folic acid to folinic acid, sequential steps in the same metabolic pathway (see Ch. 19).

6. Excretion (see p. 15)

7. Electrolyte changes
Drug-induced changes in electrolyte concentrations may influence the action of some other drugs. The best example of such an interaction is the potentiation of action of digitalis glycosides by diuretic-induced hypokalaemia.

8. Blockade of neuronal uptake
An important mechanism in the termination of action of noradrenaline is its active reuptake into noradrenergic neurones. Blockade of this reuptake process potentiates the pressor action of noradrenaline and adrenaline and of other substances that also depend on the same uptake process, such as phenylephrine. Among the groups of drugs which may block neuronal uptake are the tricyclic antidepressants (e.g. imipramine) and some adrenergic neurone blocking drugs (e.g. guanethidine, bethanidine).

Some indirectly acting sympathomimetic amines (e.g. tyramine) and some adrenergic neurone blocking drugs (e.g. guanethidine, bethanidine) depend for their pharmacological effects on being taken up into the neurone through the same uptake process as noradrenaline. Their action may, therefore, be prevented or reversed, by treatment with tricyclic antidepressant drugs.

9. Transmitter depletion

The effects of drugs which depend for their action on release of neurotransmitter substances may be reduced by the administration of other drugs which produce neurotransmitter depletion. For example, pressor responses to tyramine are reduced in reserpinised subjects.

10. Receptor blockade

The development of selective receptor blocking drugs, particularly in the autonomic nervous system and its effector organs, has led to several important clinical interactions. For example, a-adrenergic receptor blockade prevents the pressor effects of sympathomimetic amines, and β-receptor blockade reduces or abolishes their cardiac stimulating activity. Similarly, the anti-cholinergic action of several different classes of drugs (e.g. tricyclic antidepressants, antihistamines) reduces the effects of cholinomimetic agents.

11. Functional summation of effects

Drugs which produce a pharmacological effect by different biochemical mechanisms may have a synergistic interaction, for example, the mutual enhancement in the central nervous system depressant activity of anaesthetics, hypnotics, sedatives, tranquillizers and narcotic analgesics.

Other examples include the potentiation of the action of oral anticoagulant drugs by broad spectrum antibiotics which reduce vitamin K absorption, and by aspirin which inhibits prothrombin synthesis, as well as competing for plasma protein binding sites.

Catecholamines normally elevate the blood sugar level, and blockade of this effect by propranolol will potentiate the effect of oral hypoglycaemic agents.

The action of antihypertensive drugs may be increased by compounds such as alcohol which possess a general vasodilating action. On the other hand, their effects may be reduced by drugs with sodium-retaining properties such as corticosteroids and non-steroidal anti-inflammatory agents.

5

Autonomic drugs

AUTONOMIC GANGLIA

Stimulation of preganglionic nerve fibres to autonomic ganglia, both sympathetic and parasympathetic, results in the liberation of acetylcholine. Injection of very small amounts of acetylcholine into the perfusion fluid of an isolated ganglion, or into the blood supply of a ganglion produces excitation of the ganglion cells. Acetylcholinesterase is also present in the ganglia to inactivate rapidly the acetylcholine after release and receptor stimulation. This is good evidence that acetylcholine is the physiological neurotransmitter in autonomic ganglia.

The ganglionic actions of acetylcholine are referred to as its nicotinic actions, because nicotine has similar effects on autonomic ganglia. There is initial stimulation and then blockade of the ganglion cells. The effects may be summarized as:

Cardiovascular system—stimulation of sympathetic ganglia and the adrenal medulla results in release of catecholamines producing vasoconstriction, tachycardia and elevated blood pressure.

Gastrointestinal tract—initially there is increased tone and peristalsis due to parasympathetic stimulation. With higher concentrations of acetylcholine autonomic blockade occurs, with reduction of intestinal tone and motility.

Glandular secretions—initial stimulation of salivary and bronchial secretions is followed by inhibition.

Drugs blocking autonomic ganglia

It is possible to classify drugs blocking autonomic ganglia according to their mechanism of action:

(a) Depolarizing drugs, which produce a state of prolonged depolarization of the ganglion cell membrane so that the neurotransmitter cannot generate activity in the cell. Nicotine is an example of such a compound. Although of considerable pharmacological interest, depolarizing drugs have little therapeutic value as they have an initial ganglion-stimulating effect before producing blockade.

(b) Competitive blocking drugs, where the drug competes with acetylcholine for receptor sites on the ganglion cell membrane. These drugs can be further subdivided on a chemical basis:

(i) quaternary ammonium compounds, e.g. hexamethonium, pentolinium

(ii) secondary amines, e.g. mecamylamine

(iii) tertiary amines, e.g. pempidine.

Although the quaternary ammonium compounds are potent ganglion blocking agents, they are highly ionized and therefore poorly absorbed through the gastrointestinal mucous membrane. They are, therefore, unsuitable for oral administration and must be given parenterally for predictable therapeutic efficacy. Secondary amines such as mecamylamine are somewhat better absorbed, and tertiary amines, such as pempidine, are sufficiently unionized at gut pH for satisfactory blood levels to be achieved by oral administration.

Effect of autonomic ganglion blockade

Cardiovascular system—ganglionic blockade produces vasodilation, peripheral pooling of blood, decreased venous return and cardiac output, and hypotension. Under resting conditions the heart is under parasympathetic inhibitory control and blockade therefore results in tachycardia.

Gastrointestinal and urinary tracts—reduction in tone and motility produce constipation in the gut and urinary retention in the bladder.

Glandular secretions—dry mouth (xerostomia) and loss of sweating (anhidrosis) occur.

Eye—pupil dilation (mydriasis) and paralysis of accommodation.

Genital system—impotence may occur.

PERIPHERAL CHOLINERGIC NERVE TERMINAL

The actions of acetylcholine at the peripheral autonomic cholinergic nerve ending are known as its muscarinic actions, because they are mimicked by muscarine, an alkaloid derived from various species of mushroom. They may be summarized as follows:

Cardiovascular system—vasodilatation and marked slowing of the heart producing a fall in blood pressure.

Gastrointestinal tract—smooth muscles are stimulated, increasing tone and motility, with higher concentrations of acetylcholine causing spasm and tenesmus. The tone and motility of the gall bladder and bile ducts are also increased.

Glandular secretions—salivary, lachrymal, gastric, pancreatic, intestinal and mucous cells generally are stimulated.

Urogenital and respiratory tracts—smooth muscle in the bronchi, ureters and urinary bladder is stimulated leading to broncho-spasm and voiding of urine.

Eye—there is pupillary constriction, spasm of accommodation and a transitory rise in intraocular pressure followed by a more persistent fall.

Cholinomimetic drugs

Drugs mimicking the actions of acetylcholine may be divided into:

(a) Derivatives of acetylcholine e.g. methacholine, carbachol, bethanechol.

(b) Other alkaloids e.g. pilocarpine, muscarine, arecoline.

(c) Anticholinesterase drugs which inhibit or inactivate acetylcholinesterase and so allow acetylcholine to accumulate at cholinergic receptor sites and produce its effects. The most important of these are physostigmine (eserine), neostigmine (Prostigmin), pyridostigmine (Mestinon) and edrophonium (Tensilon).

Drugs blocking peripheral autonomic cholinergic junction

Parasympathetic effector organs vary in their sensitivity to the blocking effect of drugs. The most sensitive are salivary, bronchial and sweat glands which are inhibited by small concentrations. Larger doses dilate the pupils, paralyse accommodation of the eye, and block vagal tone on the heart. Still larger doses inhibit parasympathetic control of the bladder and gastrointestinal tract. Gastric secretion is the most resistant to blockade. Most drugs which block the peripheral cholinergic junction act by competitive inhibition of acetylcholine at the receptor site. This means that their action can be overcome by increasing the concentration of transmitter at the receptor site, for example by administration of an anticholinesterase drug which prevents its breakdown and allows it to accumulate until it has overcome the block.

Atropine and hyoscine

These are alkaloids derived from the belladonna plants and have been used as poisons and for medicinal purposes for thousands of years. Atropine is the racemic mixture of equal parts of D- and L-hyoscyamine, most of the antimuscarinic action residing in the

L-isomer. L-Hyoscine (scopolamine) is the active isomer, the D-isomer having no clinical importance.

The effects of atropine and hyoscine are as follows:

Eye—pupil dilatation (mydriasis) due to blockade of cholinergic tone on the sphincter pupillae. The ciliary muscle of the lens is also paralysed producing impairment of accommodation (cycloplegia) the lens being fixed for far vision. Normal pupillary reflex constriction to light or convergence is abolished. Pupil dilatation may lead to a reduction in aqueous outflow and a rise in intraocular pressure in glaucomatous patients.

Cardiovascular system—small doses of atropine slow the heart but larger doses progressively block the vagus until at a dose of about 0·04 mg/kg body weight, vagal tone is completely removed and there is a tachycardia. During the initial slowing of heart there may be disturbances of atrioventricular conduction with electrocardiographic changes.

Gastrointestinal tract—salivary secretions are inhibited producing dryness of the mouth and difficulty in talking and swallowing. There is a reduction in gut motility, and there may be associated retention of urine.

Respiratory tract—inhibition of secretion in the nose, mouth, pharynx and bronchi leads to drying of the respiratory mucous membranes. This is accompanied by a reduction in airways resistance and increase in volume of residual air.

Central nervous system—atropine and hyoscine differ in their effects on the central nervous system. Atropine stimulates the medulla and cerebral cortex leading first to increased vagal tone and respiratory activity, in higher doses to excitation, restlessness, hallucinations and delirium, and finally to medullary paralysis and death. Hyoscine, on the other hand, usually causes drowsiness and euphoria, although occasionally it may cause atropine-like excitation. It has a depressant action on vestibular function and is useful in the management of motion sickness. Both drugs have anti-tremor activity which is the basis of their use in the treatment of Parkinson's disease.

Drugs with atropine-like activity

For gastrointestinal disturbances—propantheline bromide and poldine methylsulphate reduce gastric acid secretion and are used in management of peptic ulceration. Atropine methylnitrate is used in the medical treatment of congenital hypertrophic pyloric stenosis in infants.

Mydriatics—the mydriatic effect of atropine eye drops lasts for a week or more. Homatropine hydrobromide has a more rapid action which is over in 48 hours. Eucatropine hydrochloride is another short-acting alternative with little, if any, effect on accommodation. Cyclopentolate hydrochloride has an intermediate length of action and is widely used as a mydriatic and cycloplegic agent.

Some monoamine reuptake inhibiting antidepressives—such as amitriptyline—see Chapter 7.

Antiparkinsonian drugs—see Chapter 6.

ADRENERGIC NERVE ENDING

Light and electron microscopical techniques show that sympathetic nerves end in terminal ramifications which have a beaded appearance, and fluorescent studies show that these varicosities contain granules of noradrenaline. The steps in the synthesis of noradrenaline and adrenaline are:

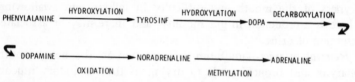

Fig. 2 Steps in the synthesis of noradrenaline and adrenaline.

Each step is controlled by enzymatic activity, but none of the enzymes is specific to adrenaline synthesis, and each takes part in other pathways. For example, L-aromatic aminoacid decarboxylase, or dopa decarboxylase, also produces 5-hydroxytryptamine and histamine from their corresponding aminoacids. The rate limiting step in this pathway is the conversion of tyrosine to dopa under the influence of tyrosine hydroxylase, and it may be blocked by certain drugs such as α-methyl paratyrosine.

Noradrenaline is found in the adrenal medulla and in the postganglionic sympathetic fibres. It disappears within a few days after nerve section. Adrenaline also is found in the adrenal medulla and in chromaffin cells elsewhere, but only insignificant amounts are found in sympathetic nerves.

It is probable that noradrenaline in sympathetic nerve terminals is in several stores or pools (Fig. 3). About 40 per cent is in the cytoplasm and the other 60 per cent is in granular stores or vesicles where it is bound to protein. It diffuses freely and passively from the granules into the cytoplasm and from the cytoplasm through the neuronal cell membrane into the extracellular space. It is car-

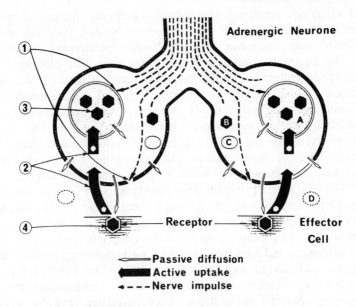

Fig. 3 Diagrammatic representation of adrenergic nerve ending and receptor.
Right: A, granular pool of noradrenaline; B, cytoplasmic pool of noradrenaline; C,
monoamine oxidase; D, catechol-*O*-methyltransferase. Left: Neurone blockade by
(1) prevention of release of noradrenaline, (2) depletion of noradrenaline stores by
prevention of uptake into neurone and into granular stores, (3) formation of false
neurotransmitter. Receptor blockade is shown at site (4). (Reproduced from P.
Turner, in *Lectures in Medicine*, 2nd edn, by C.W.H. Harvard, by kind permission
of Staples Press.)

ried in the opposite direction by active transport mechanisms from
the extracellular space into the cytoplasm, and from the cytoplasm
into the granules. Binding of noradrenaline to protein within the
granules probably represents a separate active process.

The noradrenaline in sympathetic nerve endings is, therefore,
derived from two sources:

1. Local synthesis from phenylalanine.

2. Uptake from the extracellular space of noradrenaline, released
locally, from distant sites such as the adrenal medulla, or exogenously administered. An understanding of this uptake process is
important from the point of view of inactivation of noradrenaline
after it has acted at the receptor site, for its granular binding represents a way in which it can be inactivated but used again. It
seems likely, in fact, that uptake and storage represent its major
route of inactivation under normal conditions, and that enzymatic
breakdown plays only a minor role. For this reason the excretion
rates of urinary metabolites of noradrenaline bear little relationship

to adrenergic function under normal conditions. Uptake and storage of noradrenaline are also important because they represent possible sites of action of drugs which influence adrenergic activity.

The enzymatic breakdown of noradrenaline and adrenaline is largely dependent on two enzymes, monoamine oxidase (MAO) and catechol-O-methyltransferase (COMT). MAO is widely distributed throughout the body and is concerned with the intracellular metabolism of adrenaline, noradrenaline, dopamine and 5-hydroxytryptamine. COMT is responsible for the extraneuronal metabolism of noradrenaline and adrenaline which has been released from the adrenal medulla or from sympathetic nerves.

The mechanism by which the sympathetic nerve impulse releases noradrenaline from the nerve ending is not known. In the adrenal medulla acetylcholine is liberated by preganglionic fibres and its interaction with receptors on the chromaffin cells results in release of adrenaline and noradrenaline. An intermediate step involves the entrance of calcium ions into the cells. Burn and Rand have suggested that a similar mechanism accounts for noradrenaline release from sympathetic nerve fibres. They postulated that the action potential in the postganglionic fibre causes release of acetylcholine which increases the permeability of the cell membrane to calcium ions. These enter the cell from the extracellular space and in some way promote release of noradrenaline. Although it is possible to explain the effects of many drugs on adrenergic function in terms of this unifying hypothesis, there is at present no conclusive evidence in its favour.

It is probable that the noradrenaline released by nerve impulses is that fraction in the granular or vesicular form. If so, then the release of noradrenaline from the sympathetic nerve may involve mechanisms similar to those releasing catecholamines from the adrenal medulla and chromaffin tissue elsewhere, and those releasing secretions from other cells throughout the body including insulin from the pancreas, histamine from mast cells and enzymes from digestive glands. In each case the secretion is stored in vesicles similar to those of noradrenaline in the adrenergic neurone.

Theory of stimulus secretion coupling

The theory runs as follows: the secretory product, in this case noradrenaline, is stored in subcellular granules enveloped by a membrane. Release of the substance depends on a process of exocytosis in which the full granule moves towards the periphery of the cell until the granular membrane fuses with the cell membrane under the influence of calcium ions. The cell-granular membrane then ruptures and the contents of the granule are released from the cell. The granular membrane then separates from the cell membrane and is retained for further use. The stimulus to this process varies from one type of cell to another. In the case of the neurone it is a nerve impulse, but the mechanism by which it triggers the process of exocytosis is unknown.

Presynaptic inhibition and facilitation
As well as stimulating receptors on the postsynaptic cell membrane, noradrenaline stimulates receptors on the presynaptic membrane (Fig. 4) and this acts, through a feedback mechanism, to regulate its further release. Similar mechanisms probably operate in other systems, including dopaminergic and 5-hydroxytryptaminergic neurones. Blockade of these receptors can lead either to inhibition or facilitation of transmitter release (see p. 39).

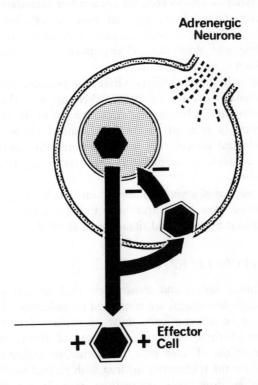

Fig. 4 Diagrammatic representation of adrenergic nerve ending and presynaptic and postsynaptic receptors. The presynaptic receptor illustrated is of inhibitory type and reduces transmitter release. Excitatory presynaptic receptors also exist (see p. 39).

SYMPATHOMIMETIC AMINES

Sympathomimetic amines, which resemble sympathetic nerve stimulation in their effects, may be divided into three groups on the basis of their mode of action.

(a) *Directly acting amines.* These have a direct action on sympathetic effector cells interacting with receptor sites on the cell membrane. They are, therefore, effective when the sympathetic nerve is depleted of its noradrenaline stores, either pharmacologically, or following sympathetic denervation. In fact, their action may be increased by such procedures to produce the phenomenon of 'denervation supersensitivity'. At least two factors seem to contribute to denervation supersensitivity. Firstly, there is a lack of the normal uptake process into the neurone, thus increasing amine concentration at the receptor site. Secondly, there appears to be an increase in the number of receptor sites, a response, presumably, of the post-synaptic cell to reduced transmitter stimulation. Most of the directly acting amines are derivatives of catechol and so are called catecholamines. They include adrenaline, noradrenaline, isoprenaline and dopamine. Phenylephrine is a directly acting amine which is not a catecholamine.

(b) *Indirectly acting amines.* These compounds, most of them non-catecholamines, act by being taken up into the adrenergic nerve ending and releasing noradrenaline on to the receptor site. Their action is reduced or abolished, therefore, by surgical or pharmacological denervation which depletes the neuronal noradrenaline content. Examples of this type are tyramine and amphetamine.

(c) *Mixed action amines.* Some amines such as ephedrine and methoxamine have both direct and indirect actions, which vary according to the species and tissue being studied.

ADRENERGIC RECEPTORS

Neurohumoral agents and transmitters such as acetylcholine and noradrenaline-like drugs, are composed of molecules. The result of their action on effector cells must be explained in terms of an interaction of these molecules, or parts of them, with specific molecules in the effector cell. The latter are called the 'specific receptors' for the transmitter or drug with respect to the particular effect. Other drug-tissue interactions that do not initiate such specific effects, such as binding of drugs to plasma proteins, binding of neurotransmitter to cell protein, and binding to enzymes for transport, storage and biotransformation are referred to in other terms such as 'secondary receptors', 'storage sites' or 'drug acceptors'.

In 1948, Ahlquist suggested that the effects of adrenaline at peripheral sympathetic sites could be divided into two groups with two types of postsynaptic receptor, α and β . These were originally called excitatory and inhibitory receptors, respectively, because of their general tendency to produce excitation or inhibition when stimulated, but as there are important exceptions to this in both groups it is proposed to refer to them as α or β-receptors. Further investigations have shown that the β-group can be subdivided into β_1 and β_2-receptors. Important receptor actions and examples of compounds which selectively activate or block these receptors are given in Table 5. Adrenaline has both α and β actions and its effects will be the result of summation of these actions when they are interrelated.

Presynaptic receptors (see p. 37) appear to be of both α - and β -type; the latter possess a low threshold for stimulation and cause facilitation of noradrenaline release, while the α-receptors have a higher threshold and inhibit release. This may be seen as a regulatory mechanism, at first amplifying the transmitter action and then terminating it. Presynaptic α-receptor blockade will, of course, facilitate transmitter release while β-blockade will inhibit it.

It is probable that the adrenergic receptor is linked to the enzyme adenylcyclase which catalyses the conversation of ATP to cyclic AMP (Fig. 5), and so is responsible for initiating the appropriate biological effects.

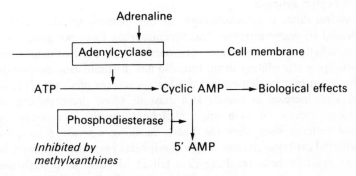

Fig. 5 The relationship of adenylcyclase to adrenaline activity.

Cyclic AMP is inactivated by conversion to 5' AMP under the influence of the enzyme phosphodiesterase. This enzyme can itself

Table 5

Receptor	Selectively activated by	Selectively blocked by	Main actions of receptor stimulation
	Noradrenaline	Phenoxybenzamine	Vasoconstriction of skin, splanchnic and coronary vessels
	Phenylephrine	Phentolamine	Pupil dilatation
	Methoxamine	Thymoxamine	Relaxation of gut
		Indoramin	Bronchoconstriction
			Hyperglycaemia and increase in plasma FFA
	Dobutamine		Increased inotropic and chronotropic cardiac action
		Acebutolol	
		Atenolol	
		Metoprolol	
	Alprenolol	Practolol	
	Nadolol		
	Oxprenolol		
	Pindolol		
	Fenoterol	Propranolol	
	Isoetharine	Sotalol	Vasodilation of coronary, skeletal muscle and some skin vessels
	Orciprenaline	Timolol	
	Rimiterol		Bronchial relaxation
	Salbutamol		Tremor
	Terbutaline		Relaxation of uterus
			Hyperglycaemia and increase in plasma FFA*

*It is uncertain, at present, in which of the β-receptor subdivisions these actions should be included.

be inhibited by drugs of the methylxanthine group such as caffeine and theophylline, the effects of which, therefore, mimic sympathetic stimulation in many ways.

α-receptor agonists

Noradrenaline, a catecholamine, is the neurochemical mediator released by nerve impulses and various drugs from postganglionic sympathetic or 'adrenergic' neurones. It is predominantly an α-receptor stimulating drug, but also has β-stimulating properties which can best be demonstrated after α-receptor blockade. It produces an increase in systolic and diastolic blood pressures due to vasoconstriction of skin and splanchnic vessels. Compensatory vagal reflexes then slow the heart, masking a weak β-receptor mediated cardioaccelerator action. Peripheral resistance increases in most vascular beds resulting in a fall in blood flow through the kidney, brain, liver and splanchnic regions. Indications for its use are conditions of serious hypotension, but it must be emphasized that any increase in blood pressure produced by noradrenaline is at the expense of tissue perfusion. Toxic effects are the result of its pressor action and include headache, photophobia and vomiting, and the serious consequences of hypertension such as cerebral haemorrhage and pulmonary oedema.

Phenylephrine is a powerful α-receptor stimulating drug with only little β-receptor activity. Its effects on the cardiovascular system are similar to those of noradrenaline on α-receptors, with hypertension due to widespread vasoconstriction leading to reflex bradycardia. Renal and skin blood flows are reduced. Its absorption from the gastrointestinal tract is unreliable, and it is an unsatisfactory and inconsistent mydriatic, except in the presence of denervation where it produces a potentiated mydriasis. It is used in several nasal decongestant preparations because of its vasoconstrictor action.

β-receptor agonists

Isoprenaline is a catecholamine with potent β-receptor stimulating properties. It also has weak α-receptor stimulating properties, but these can only be shown on certain organs in the presence of β-blockade. It is a general β-stimulant and is not selective in its action on β_1 or β_2-receptors.

Cardiovascular effects. Isoprenaline increases cardiac output by positive inotropic and chronotropic actions, that is, it increases both the force and rate of myocardial contractions. It dilates coronary and skeletal muscle arteries, and to a lesser extent renal, mesenteric and skin blood vessels. This results in a fall in diastolic blood pressure, but because of the increased cardiac output, mean blood pressure may not fall to the same extent.

Respiratory system. Isoprenaline stimulates the respiratory centre, increasing the rate and depth of respiration. It is a potent bronchodilator, stimulating β-receptors in the bronchial musculature, and this is the basis for its widespread clinical use in bronchial asthma.

Other smooth muscle. Isoprenaline decreases the tone and motility of the musculature of the gastrointestinal tract, and inhibits uterine motility and tone.

Central nervous system. Isoprenaline produces central nervous stimulation with anxiety, restlessness and vomiting. Psychological dependence may develop in asthmatic patients treated for long periods with aerosol preparations. It also increases tremor and the rate of muscle contraction in reflexes.

Isoprenaline is absorbed sublingually and by aerosol but its absorption from the gastrointestinal tract is unpredictable.

Unwanted effects include palpitations, tachycardia, dysrhythmias and anginal pain. Administration of large doses over long periods of time may produce myocardial necrosis in experimental animals.

Salbutamol is a sympathomimetic amine which acts preferentially on β_2-receptors to produce bronchodilatation and vasodilatation of skeletal muscle arterioles in doses which do not produce a significant increase in rate and force of cardiac contraction. In higher doses, however, cardiac effects are seen and tremor occurs. It is widely used in the treatment of bronchial asthma and is administered by inhalation, intravenous infusion or in tablet form.

Fenoterol, isoetharine, rimiterol and terbutaline are other selective β_2-agonists with similar properties to salbutamol.

Indications for β_2-agonists
1. Bronchial asthma (see Ch. 11).
2. Cardiac failure and heart block (see Ch. 8).
3. Premature labour (see Ch. 15).

Adrenaline
Adrenaline is produced by cells of the adrenal medulla and chromaffin tissue elsewhere in the body. It stimulates both α and β-adrenergic receptors throughout the body, its effects on different organs depending on the distribution of receptors within them.

Cardiovascular system. Adrenaline has a direct stimulating action on the heart mediated through its β-receptors, increasing the strength of ventricular contraction and the heart rate, and dilating coronary vessels. The response of blood vessels to adrenaline varies according to their α and β-receptor distribution. Arteriolar vessels in skin, mucosa and kidney are generally constricted by the action of α-receptors, but there are some vessels which dilate due to β-receptor stimulation in certain regions. Arterioles in skeletal muscles are dilated due to their β-receptors. The vasoconstrictor effects therefore tend to increase systemic blood pressure while the dilatation of skeletal vessels tends to decrease it.

Gastrointestinal tract. Its effects on the gut depend on initial tone and motility, but in general are to reduce tone and contract the pyloric and ileocaecal sphincters.

Respiratory system. Adrenaline has a brief stimulant effect on the respiratory centre, but this is not of therapeutic value. Its main effects are on β-receptors in the bronchial musculature producing relaxation which is most evident when the muscle is contracted due to disease such as bronchial asthma, to vagal stimulation or to drugs such as histamine or cholinergic agents. It also produces vasoconstriction in the bronchial mucosa to reduce vascularity and engorgement.

Eye. It has little effect on the pupil when applied locally, but in the sympathectomized eye, or following treatment with local guanethidine it produces marked mydriasis. Adrenaline lowers intraocular pressure in normal subjects and in glaucoma.

As adrenaline is rapidly destroyed in the gastrointestinal tract it must be given parenterally by the intramuscular or subcutaneous routes, or by inhalation.

Therapeutic uses

(a) Cardiac arrest.

(b) Urticaria, angioneurotic oedema and serum sickness, when its subcutaneous administration gives prompt and dramatic relief.

(c) In combination with local anaesthetics to limit their rate of absorption and provide a bloodless field of operation.

(d) Its use in bronchial asthma has been superseded by β_2-selective stimulant drugs.

Toxicity

The chief toxic effect of adrenaline is acute hypertension with its complications, particularly pulmonary oedema. Cardiac dysrhythmias may also occur, particularly during anaesthesia with halogenated hydrocarbon anaesthetics such as chloroform and halothane.

ADRENERGIC NEURONE AND RECEPTOR BLOCKADE

Adrenergic neurone blockade

Blockade of adrenergic neurone activity may be achieved in three ways (Fig. 3).

(a) The release of noradrenaline by a nerve impulse is prevented, although noradrenaline depletion does not occur.

(b) Noradrenaline depletion occurs so that there is none available for release by a nerve impulse.

(c) Noradrenaline synthesis is impaired, or a false transmitter is substituted for noradrenaline with a weaker pressor action, so that sympathetic nerve activity results in a reduced pressor response.

Guanethidine

Guanethidine specifically blocks adrenergic neurone activity, by two distinct mechanisms.

(a) It prevents the release of noradrenaline in response to sympathetic nerve stimulation, even though noradrenaline stores remain intact. It is probable that this is the mechanism of its action responsible for its antihypertensive effect in therapeutic doses, for indirectly-acting amines such as tyramine still possess pressor and mydriatic activity in hypertensive patients treated with oral guanethidine.

(b) Higher concentrations of guanethidine, achieved for example by intravenous administration, produce depletion of noradrenaline from the adrenergic neurone by a release process which may result in an initial hypertensive effect before the blood pressure falls. Similarly, the local instillation of guanethidine into the eye results in an initial mydriasis due to noradrenaline release before the appearance of miosis.

As with ganglion-blocking drugs, the antihypertensive effect depends on peripheral pooling with reduced venous return and cardiac output. Patients should be treated as far as possible in the upright posture rather than supine, and should be advised to avoid sudden changes in position and rate of movement to reduce the risk of postural hypotension. Guanethidine has a long half-life in the body and its action is slow to develop. It is administered in a single daily dose starting with 10 to 20 mg and increments should not be given more frequently than every 4 to 7 days. Tolerance may develop.

The commonest side-effects of treatment are diarrhoea and parotid pain. Nasal congestion, muscular weakness, fluid retention and failure of ejaculation may be troublesome. Rarely guanethidine produces mental depression.

Bethanidine

This antihypertensive drug has similar pharmacological properties to guanethidine, but is more rapidly excreted and its effects are therefore much shorter. It is administered in divided daily doses every 6 to 8 hours. Postural hypotension and the other side-effects of treatment with guanethidine may also be seen with bethanidine.

Debrisoquine

Like guanethidine and bethanidine in oral doses, debrisoquine produces adrenergic neurone blockade without noradrenaline depletion. Intravenous debrisoquine, however, produces a sharp rise in blood pressure, which is probably due to release of nor-adrenaline from adrenergic nerve endings. Side-effects are similar to those observed with guanethidine and bethanidine.

Reserpine

Reserpine is an alkaloid obtained from the roots of *Rauwolfia serpentina*, a climbing shrub indigenous to India and neighbouring countries. It depletes tissues of noradrenaline, 5-hydroxytryptamine and dopamine. While its central tranquillizing activity is probably associated with changes in concentration of these amines in the brain, its antihypertensive effect is due largely to depletion of noradrenaline from adrenergic nerve endings in the heart and blood vessels. This leads to vasodilatation, reduced venous return and diminished cardiac output, while vagal predominance in the heart produces bradycardia.

The most serious side-effect of treatment with reserpine is mental depression which may be severe enough to cause suicidal attempts by some patients. This is seen particularly if the daily dose exceeds 0·3 mg, but successful antihypertensive therapy can usually be achieved by doses between 0·1 and 0·25 mg daily, given in a single oral dose because of its cumulative effect.

Depletion of brain dopamine by reserpine in large doses may produce Parkinsonism accompanied by choreoathetosis and cerebellar ataxia, and hyperprolactinaemia with galactorrhoea. Diarrhoea, nasal stuffiness, fluid retention with cardiac failure, and endocrine disturbances such as amenorrhoea, gynaecomastia, and impairment of sexual function have been described. Increased gastric secretion may lead to reactivation of peptic ulcer with the complications of haemorrhage and perforation. A report of an increased incidence of carcinoma of the breast in women treated with reserpine for hypertension has not been confirmed in several studies involving larger numbers of patients.

α-Methyldopa

The mechanism of action of α-methyldopa is still obscure. It both inhibits the synthesis of noradrenaline and is itself converted into a false transmitter, α-methylnoradrenaline, which replaces noradrenaline in the sympathetic nerve ending. However, pharmacological studies with α-methylnoradrenaline in man and on human tissues have not provided conclusive evidence that it is a weaker pressor agent than noradrenaline. Indeed, there is evidence in animals that α-methylnoradrenaline is a more potent agonist than noradrenaline at central adrenergic α-receptors which regulate sympathetic outflow (p. 56); stimulation of these receptors leads to a reduction in peripheral sympathetic tone. Premedication with a selective α-receptor blocking drug such as phentolamine prevents this action.

Whereas the effects of guanethidine, bethanidine and debrisoquine are seen predominantly in the erect position, with postural hypotension as a common side-effect of treatment, α-methyldopa reduces blood pressure in both recumbent and upright positions.

The most common side-effect of treatment with α-methyldopa is sedation, probably due to depletion of noradrenaline from the brain. It tends to disappear with continued administration of the drug, but withdrawal of treatment after a long period of administration may result in the appearance of a state of excitement with restlessness and insomnia. Like the other adrenergic neurone-blocking drugs it may cause bradycardia, stuffy nose, failure of ejaculation, and sodium and water retention with oedema and cardiac failure. A positive antiglobulin (Coomb's) test has been found in 20 per cent of patients taking α-methyldopa, but clinical evidence of haemolysis is rare.

ADRENERGIC RECEPTOR BLOCKADE

Drugs which prevent or interfere with the release of noradrenaline from the adrenergic neurone block sympathetic activity irrespective of whether the nerve is supplying α or β-receptors and the result is a general reduction in sympathetic activity. Those now to be discussed act at the receptor site, blocking the effects of noradrenaline and other directly-acting amines on either α or β-receptors. In general, they are more effective against circulating catecholamines than against those endogenously derived from neurotransmitter stores in the body.

α-Adrenergic receptor blocking drugs

Phenoxybenzamine and dibenamine
These drugs are chemically related to the nitrogen mustards and are alkylating agents. They are highly reactive and have other pharmacological actions than simple α-adrenergic receptor blockade, including blockade of histamine and 5-hydroxytryptamine on smooth muscle. Small doses produce sedation probably due to their α-adrenergic blocking action, but high doses produce central nervous stimulation with nausea, vomiting, hyperventilation and convulsions.

The effects of α-adrenergic receptor blockade in therapeutic doses are chiefly seen in the cardiovascular system, where a small fall in diastolic pressure occurs with a compensatory tachycardia. If the plasma volume is reduced, however, or if hypertension is present, a marked fall in blood pressure may occur, which is greater in the erect than supine position. These drugs may be administered orally or parenterally and adrenergic blockade may persist for up to 3 to 4 days.

Tolazoline
This is a competitive inhibitor of α-adrenergic receptor activity, and also of 5-hydroxytryptamine. In addition it has a direct relaxant action on smooth muscle and intrinsic sympathomimetic (partial agonist) activity including cardiac stimulation. It has cholinergic effects on the gastrointestinal tract which are blocked by atropine, and histamine-like actions such as stimulation of gastric secretion. Its effects on the cardiovascular system are, therefore, complex and depend on several types of action. Side effects include flushing, tachycardia, dysrhythmias, anginal pain, nausea, vomiting, diarrhoea and exacerbation of peptic ulcer.

Phentolamine
Phentolamine resembles tolazoline in possessing other marked pharmacological effects besides its α-receptor blocking properties. In particular it has potent smooth muscle relaxing effects, and intrinsic sympathomimetic activity. The first may lead to a profound reduction in blood pressure and so produce a false positive in the 'Rogitine test' for diagnosis of a phaeochromocytoma. This test depends on producing a fall in blood pressure with intravenous phentolamine in patients in whom hypertension is due to a phaeochromocytoma. It has, however, been superseded by direct measurement of urinary or plasma catecholamines or their metabolites. The intrinsic sympathomimetic activity includes cardiac stimulation, and palpitations and tachycardia may be distressing following intravenous administration. Other side-effects include nasal congestion, nausea, vomiting and diarrhoea.

Thymoxamine
Thymoxamine is a competitive α-receptor blocking drug with relatively few other important pharmacological actions, which include weak antihistamine effects. It produces miosis when applied locally to the eye, and a rise in skin temperature when applied in a water-free cetomacrogol base, due to reduction in α-receptor-mediated vasoconstriction in the skin leading to an increase in cutaneous blood flow. A fall in systemic blood pressure, particularly marked in the erect position, occurs after intravenous administration, and also after large oral doses. It has a very short plasma half-life, however, and its absorption after oral administration is erratic.

Indoramin

This has recently been introduced as an antihypertensive drug. Its action in therapeutic doses appears to depend largely on α-receptor blockade although in higher concentrations myocardial depression may occur. It also has antihistamine properties. Sedation commonly occurs.

Prazosin

When first introduced as an antihypertensive agent, prazosin was thought to act primarily through direct smooth muscle relaxation. It is now believed to be a competitive α-adrenoceptor blocking drug which also possesses some direct relaxant properties. It lowers blood pressure by producing dilatation particularly of resistance arterioles. Dizziness and headaches may occur with its use, but its most important adverse effect is a transient loss of consciousness associated with profound hypotension which, while it most commonly occurs at the start of treatment, may also occur at other times, and the exact cause of which is not yet understood. Patients treated with prazosin should be kept under observation for some hours after receiving the first dose, which should always be small.

Ergot

Ergot alkaloids were the first adrenergic blocking drugs to be discovered by the classical studies of Dale in 1906. Most of their pharmacological and therapeutic actions are due to properties other than adrenergic blockade, however, and the true nature of their activity is not yet known in detail. They have a direct stimulant action on smooth muscle, which may in fact be a sympathomimetic action. This is responsible for the rise in blood pressure which ergot preparations produce, and for the coronary vasoconstriction which may occur and cause marked ischaemia in patients with coronary artery disease. Prolonged administration may cause vascular insufficiency and gangrene of the extremities.

Indications for α-*receptor blockade*

Although α-adrenergic receptor blocking drugs are widely prescribed for a variety of conditions, their proven value is limited to a few well-defined situations.

(a) *Phaeochromocytoma*. While of doubtful value in the diagnosis of this condition, α-receptor blockade is indicated in the preoperative and operative management of the established case, where it prevents the paroxysmal hypertension which characterizes the condition and which is particularly likely to occur during operative manipulation of the tumour. Phenoxybenzamine is most often used, and is given orally preoperatively and intravenously for 12 hours before and during surgery.

(b) *Essential Hypertension*. Phenoxybenzamine and phentolamine have little place in the management of essential hypertension, largely due to their other unwanted and unpleasant pharmacological actions. Prazosin, however, is now established in the management of hypertensive patients who have not been controlled with combined diuretic + β-adrenoceptor blocking drug or diuretic + methyldopa treatment, and in whom the addition of prazosin may produce a further fall in blood pressure. Any reflex tachycardia that might accompany its vasodilating effects will be reduced or prevented by the accompanying administration of a β-receptor blocking drug. Indoramin may also prove to be an effective antihypertensive agent, although its sedative properties may be a limitation to its use. Reflex tachycardia seldom appears to be associated with its antihypertensive action.

(c) *Shock*. In the past it has been part of the standard treatment of cardiovascular shock to administer sympathomimetic pressor agents such as noradrenaline to increase blood pressure, even though the effect of these drugs has been to reduce blood flow to organs such as the kidneys and gut. This is particularly dangerous in conditions such as haemorrhage, trauma or infection where hypovolaemia may be present. There is evidence that the best way to treat such conditions is to induce vasodilatation by inhibiting sympathetic vasoconstriction with α-receptor blocking drugs or by directly relaxing vascular smooth muscle, together with expansion of the plasma volume with blood or other suitable fluids.

(d) *Peripheral vascular disease*. Although the α-receptor blocking drugs phenoxybenzamine, tolazoline and thymoxamine have been widely used in peripheral vascular disease, their real value has yet to be established. There is evidence that in intermittent claudication blood may actually be shunted away from the ischaemic limb to normal areas because of vasodilatation in them. Vasodilatation in skeletal muscle arterioles is β-receptor mediated, and it is therefore unlikely that α-receptor blocking drugs would be effective in claudication. On theoretical grounds ischaemic conditions of the skin are the most likely form of peripheral vascular disease to be helped by these drugs, but confirmation in clinical trials is not yet available.

(e) *Cardiac failure*. A recent development in the treatment of cardiac failure resistant to diuretic-digitalis therapy has been the use of drugs which reduce the preload and afterload on the left ventricle. Preload reduction may be achieved by veno-dilatation by the cautious use of nitrates such as isosorbide dinitrate (p. 134). Afterload reduction is achieved by reducing the resistance to left ventricular ejection by an arteriolar vasodilator such as phentolamine, prazosin or hydralazine (see p. 58). Although these drugs also have some effect on the venous side, the fall in filling pressure is more than compensated by the reduction in afterload, and cardiac output tends to rise rather than fall. As a result of increased stroke volume, mean blood pressure may not fall.

β-Adrenergic receptor blocking drugs

In general, β-adrenergic receptor blocking drugs are structurally similar to the β-adrenergic agonist drugs such as isoprenaline. The first of this class to be introduced was dichloroisoprenaline (DCI) which blocked those responses to adrenaline and other sympathomimetic amines which involve β-receptors, but also had intrinsic agonist activity of its own comparable to that of isoprenaline. As a result it was not of clinical value. Pronethalol was more suitable for clinical use as it had considerably less intrinsic activity than DCI, but repeated administration to mice over a long period of time appeared to have carcinogenic effects and it was, therefore, withdrawn.

There are now several potent β-receptor blocking drugs which differ in certain properties such as partial agonist (or intrinsic sympathomimetic) activity, membrane stabilizing activity, and selectivity of action at different β-receptors (Table 6). In general, however, they have the following effects:

Table 6 Comparative properties of β-adrenoceptor blocking drugs.

Drug	Selectivity for B_1 receptors	Partial agonist activity	Membrane stabilising activity
Acebutolol	+	+	+
Alprenolol	−	+	+
Atenolol	+	−	−
Metoprolol	+	−	−
Nadolol	−	−	−
Oxprenolol	−	+	+
Pindolol	−	+	+
Practolol	+	+	−
Propranolol	−	−	+
Sotalol	−	−	−
Timolol	−	?	−

(a) *Cardiovascular system.* β-receptor blocking drugs, such as propranolol, produce a fall in heart rate, cardiac output, arterial pressure and left ventricular minute work, and also increase the systolic and diastolic transverse diameters of the heart. During exercise the effects are much greater, with reduction of the normal increment of heart rate, cardiac output, mean arterial pressure and left ventricular minute work, and an increase in the arterio-mixed venous oxygen difference. Propranolol is a racemic mixture of (+)- and (−)-isomers, and it appears that the β-receptor blocking properties reside predominantly in the (−) isomer. In higher concentrations propranolol has direct membrane-stabilizing or 'quinidine-like' effects on the myocardium.

(b) *Respiratory system.* Sympathetically induced bronchodilatation is mediate by the β-adrenergic receptors, and their blockade by β-blocking drugs may, therefore, lead to an increase in airways resistance. This may be particularly harmful to patients with bronchial asthma, chronic bronchitis, or other forms of respiratory insufficiency. A number of β-blocking drugs have been developed which appear to possess certain degrees of selectivity of action, blocking β_1-receptors in the heart (p. 40) at lower concentrations than the β_2-receptors in the bronchi. Practolol is the most cardioselective of these drugs, but has had to be withdrawn from general clinical use because it has produced a syndrome comprising psoriasiform rashes, dry eyes progressing to more serious ophthalmic changes, and sclerosing peritonitis, sometimes associated with antinuclear factor. Acebutolol, atenolol and metoprolol are other 'cardioselective' drugs which are in therapeutic use. Their cardioselectivity is, however, only relative, and in the oral therapeutic doses normally used in hypertension and angina, they may produce clinically important increases in airways resistance. Their advantage over non-selective drugs such as alprenolol, nadolol, propranolol, oxprenolol, pindolol, sotalol and timolol appears to be that their bronchoconstricting action can be more readily overcome by administration of a β_2 agonist drug such as rimiterol, salbutamol or terbutaline. Some β-blocking drugs, including alprenolol, oxprenolol and pindolol are partial agonists, having a receptor stimulant as well as blocking action, and there is evidence that this property may confer some advantage over drugs without it in patients with asthma. However, it must be emphasized that all β-blocking drugs may precipitate asthmatic attacks in patients with this condition, and they are, therefore, contraindicated in such patients.

(c) *Nervous system*. There is evidence that the central control of blood pressure is influenced by central α- and β-adrenoceptor activity, stimulation of central α-receptors producing a fall in blood pressure, and stimulation of central β₁-receptors a rise in blood pressure. Central β-blockade might, therefore, produce a fall in sympathetic outflow and systemic blood pressure (p. 56), but there is little evidence that this contributes to the antihypertensive effect of β-blocking drugs. Central nervous adverse effects occur quite frequently with these drugs, however, including sleep disturbances, dreams, hypnogogic hallucinations, lethargy, sedation and depression. Propranolol has also been claimed to possess anti-psychotic effects in high doses such as 1–2 g daily, about ten times the usual dose for other indications. Such central actions are not necessarily due to β-receptor blockade, for these drugs also possess potent central 5HT antagonist properties which might account for some of these effects. Furthermore, brain cell concentrations of propranolol achieved with the high doses of propranolol used in antipsychotic treatment might be associated with direct membrane-stabilising activity.

Isoprenaline and adrenaline increase tremor by a direct action on skeletal muscle, and this may be prevented by β-receptor blocking drugs, although it is uncertain whether this is entirely due to peripheral blockade or whether there is a central component to their anti-tremor action. It appears that tremor is mediated mainly through β₂-receptors.

(d) *Eye*. Some β-blocking drugs, such as propranolol, which possess local anaesthetic properties produce marked corneal anaesthesia when instilled into the eye, and have been used surgically for this purpose.

Intraocular pressure may, paradoxically, be reduced by both α-and β-adrenoceptor agonists and antagonists because of their different actions on aqueous production and reabsorption. Most β-blocking drugs reduce intraocular pressure, at least transiently, and timolol appears to have a sustained ocular hypotensive action which is being widely exploited in the treatment of glaucoma. Even when timolol is instilled into the conjunctival sac for this purpose, however, sufficient may be absorbed systemically to produce the cardiovascular and other effects of β-receptor blockade.

Drugs with both α- and β-receptor blocking properties

It is possible that some β-blocking drugs possess minor α-adrenoceptor blocking properties. Labetalol, however, combines α-and β-receptor blocking activity in a ratio of about 1:5 and is an effective antihypertensive agent, particularly when used intravenously to control severe hypertension. Adverse effects include postural hypotension, bronchoconstriction, nasal stuffiness, vivid dreams, epigastric pain and itching of the scalp.

Indications for β-receptor blockade

(a) *Angina*. Coronary vasodilatation is mediated by β-receptor activity, and β-blockade may produce a fall in coronary flow. However, the reduction in cardiac work and oxygen requirements which it produces, particularly during exercise or emotional states, may be greater than its effects on coronary flow, and so the use of propranolol and other β-blocking drugs has proved to be of value in many cases of angina pectoris. Large doses are required in many patients, however, in excess of those needed to block exogenously administered isoprenaline, and it is possible, therefore, that other mechanisms of action may be involved.

(b) *Cardiac dysrhythmias*. β-Receptor blocking drugs prevent or abolish catecholamine-induced dysrhythmias in experimental animals and man, and are of value in the management of patients with phaeochromocytoma at risk from ventricular dysrhythmias. They may also abolish digitalis-induced dysrhythmias, the mechanism of this being uncertain.

(c) *Hypertension*. β-Receptor blocking drugs have significant antihypertensive effects which may be seen when used alone or in combination with other antihypertensive drugs or thiazide diuretics. This action is not yet fully understood, but may involve several factors including (1) blockade of central β-receptors involved in blood pressure control and sympathetic outflow (p. 56): (2) inhibition of renin production in the kidney, which is mediated, at least in part, by β-adrenergic activity, with an associated fall in angiotensin generation and aldosterone secretion: (3) a fall in cardiac output, although this may be followed by a reflex increase in peripheral resistance: (4) an influence on baroreceptor activity. (5) blockade of presynaptic β-receptors may lead to a decrease of noradrenaline release in response to sympathetic nervous activity and therefore to a reduction in postsynaptic adrenoceptor stimulation (p. 39).

(d) *Hypertrophic cardiomyopathy*. In this disease there is a subaortic stenosis which worsens whenever myocardial contractility increases, as for example, from increased sympathetic activity associated with exercise or emotion. β-Blocking drugs have been shown to reduce or prevent this, and have proved of value in the management of patients with this condition, reducing the frequency of anginal attacks and dyspnoea which characterize it. They have also been shown to reduce the frequency and severity of dyspnoeic attacks in Fallot's tetralogy, again by decreasing contractility and the constriction of right ventricular outflow which accompanies it.

(e) *Phaeochromocytoma*. When α-receptors are blocked with phenoxybenzamine, catecholamines produced by the tumour can still produce an increase in heart rate or a dysrhythmia by β-receptor stimulation. This occurs irrespective of whether adrenaline or noradrenaline is the predominant catecholamine secreted by the tumour. These effects can be prevented or abolished by a β-receptor blocking drug such as propranolol, given by mouth in the preoperative period after commencement of treatment with an α-receptor blocking drug, and intravenously during operative removal of the tumour.

(f) *Hyperthyroidism*. Many of the peripheral manifestations of hyperthyroidism are due to increased β-receptor activity and may be reduced by β-blocking drugs. In this condition there is also increased responsiveness to adrenergic stimulation, however, and therefore those drugs which possess intrinsic agonist activity are not so effective as those without it such as propranolol and sotalol.

(g) *Anxiety*. Autonomic activity, particularly sympathetic, is prominent in anxiety states, and propranolol has been shown to significantly reduce the physical symptomatology of patients with this condition. Its effects are particularly seen where complaints of palpitations and tachycardia are prominent, but may also relieve other autonomic effects such as sweating and diarrhoea.

(h) *Tremor*. β-blocking drugs reduce both physiological and essential tremor by a direct action on skeletal muscle. This is probably a β_2-mediated effect.

(i) *Psychosis*. Some uncontrolled studies have suggested that propranolol may have therapeutic effects in the psychosis associated with porphyria and the post-partum state, and in schizophrenia. The pharmacological basis of this action, which awaits confirmation in controlled trials, is not known although there is animal evidence that propranolol may inhibit central 5-hydroxytryptamine activity.

(j) *Glaucoma* (see p. 52)

Untoward effects of β-receptor blockade
(a) *Cardiovascular*. β-blocking drugs may precipitate or make worse cardiac failure, due to withdrawal of cardiac sympathetic drive, and they should be used with great caution in patients with reduced cardiac reserve. They may also exacerbate Raynaud's

phenomenon and produce cold extremities, due to unopposed cutaneous α-receptor vasoconstriction.

(b) *Respiratory*. These have already been discussed (p. 51).

(c) *Central nervous*. Sleep disturbance, nightmares, hallucinations, and depression occur rarely (p. 52).

(d) *Others*. Potentiation of the hypoglycaemic action of insulin and sulphonylurea antidiabetic drugs may occur. The practolol syndrome which lead to its withdrawal has already been discussed (p. 51).

HYPERTENSION

The role of adrenergic receptor blocking drugs in the treatment of phaeochromocytoma has already been discussed. In forms of hypertension due to other known pathological causes, and in essential hypertension, drugs which influence sympathetic control of the

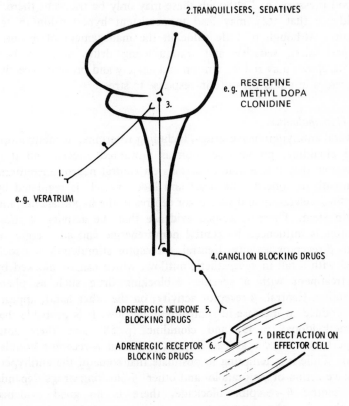

Fig. 6 Sites at which drugs may interfere with sympathetic activity.

heart and blood vessels, and drugs which influence vascular tone by other mechanisms may be effective in reducing blood pressure, even though increased sympathetic tone may not be primarily responsible for the condition. Sites at which drugs may interfere with sympathetic activity in the management of hypertension are shown in Figure 6.

1. The afferent neurone

The veratrum alkaloids interfere with afferent autonomic neurone activity, particularly from pressure and stretch receptors in the heart and carotid-sinus baroreceptor areas, resulting in a reduction in sympathetic outflow from the hypothalamus. They have marked toxic effects, however, and are not used clinically.

2. Cortical function

Anxiety and emotional stress may be associated with increases in blood pressure, and although these may only be transient there is evidence that they may lead to persistent hypertension in the future. Although of little value in the management of essential hypertension, sedative and tranquillizing drugs such as benzodiazepines may reduce tension and anxiety and prevent excessive increases in blood pressure in response to stress.

3. Hypothalamus

Several antihypertensive drugs, including reserpine, α-methyldopa and clonidine, produce sedation as unwanted effects, and it is probable that this is due to actions on central neurotransmitters. Sympathetic tone on the heart and blood vessels is regulated by cardio-acceleratory and vasomotor centres in the hypothalamus and brain stem. There is animal evidence that the activity of these centres is influenced by central noradrenergic and adrenergic α- and β-receptor activity. Central α-receptor stimulation is associated with a fall in sympathetic outflow, which can be blocked by pretreatment with a specific α-blocking drug such as phentolamine. Central β-receptor activity, on the other hand, appears to produce an increase in sympathetic outflow. It is probable that α-methyldopa (p. 45) and clonidine (p. 58) owe their antihypertensive effects, at least in part, to central α-receptor stimulation. While it is tempting to postulate that some of the antihypertensive action of propranolol and other β-blocking drugs depends on central β-receptor blockade, there is no good evidence for this.

4. Autonomic ganglia

Drugs blocking autonomic ganglia have already been discussed. Because of their erratic absorption from the gut, and the unpleasant effects of general autonomic blockade which they produce, their use is restricted to the treatment of hypertensive emergencies, where they are administered parenterally until the blood pressure is brought under control.

5. Adrenergic neurone

The actions of guanethidine, bethanidine, debrisoquine and reserpine have already been discussed (pp. 43–45). Their use is decreasing, largely because of their adverse effects and the important interactions of the first three with monoamine reuptake inhibiting drugs (p. 28).

6. Adrenergic receptor

α-adrenergic receptor blocking drugs are useful in the management of phaeochromocytoma. Although earlier non-competitive drugs, such as phenoxybenzamine, have little place in essential hypertension, the competitive α-blocking drug prazosin appears to be of value in some patients with essential hypertension who have failed to respond adequately to first-line treatment (p. 48). β-receptor blocking drugs are now considered by many physicians to be the firstline treatment in essential hypertension as well as in protecting the myocardium from the effects of excess catecholamines in patients with phaeochromocytomata. Labetalol, which combines α- and β-adrenoceptor blocking activity (p. 52) is particularly valuable when administered intravenously in management of severely hypertensive patients.

7. Drugs acting directly on the vascular smooth muscle

(a) Thiazide diuretics and other related compounds such as indapamide have an antihypertensive action which may be effective in sub-diuretic doses and does not appear to depend simply on reduction in extracellular fluid volume and cardiac output. They may have a direct action on the blood vessel wall, reducing its sensitivity to catecholamines, angiotensin and other pressor substances by mechanisms beyond the adrenoceptor. They may be used alone in the management of essential hypertension, or may be used together with other drugs such as β-antagonists, α-methyldopa and more potent vasodilators. The doses of the latter may, therefore, be reduced with a consequent reduction in incidence of adverse effects and cost of treatment. Plasma potassium concentrations should be monitored in patients requiring digitalis treatment for atrial fibrillation or cardiac failure (p. 126).

Diazoxide is a thiazide drug without diuretic activity, but with marked hyperglycaemic and hypotensive effects. It is given by intravenous administration in acute hypertensive emergencies while treatment with an oral agent is substituted.

(b) Hydralazine probably owes its antihypertensive action predominantly to a generalised direct relaxation of vascular smooth muscle. It became unpopular because of its undesirable effects, the most common being headache, palpitations, tachycardia, angina, anorexia, nausea and vomiting. More dangerous are bone marrow depression, an acute rheumatoid state, and rarely, a syndrome resembling systemic lupus erythematosus. However, it has regained some popularity as a second-line treatment of essential hypertension in patients already receiving a β-adrenoceptor blocking drug together with a thiazide-type drug but with inadequate blood pressure control. The addition of relatively small doses of hydralazine may achieve satisfactory levels of blood pressure with little risk of adverse effects, tachycardia and angina seldom occurring in the presence of β-blockade.

(c) Minoxidil is a highly-potent vasodilator which may be effective in patients whose blood pressure has not been controlled with other drugs. Its major adverse effect is increased hair growth which can be distressing particularly in women.

(d) Clonidine is a potent antihypertensive drug whose mode of action is not yet clearly understood. While there is some evidence for a central action (p. 56), it has peripheral effects on blood vessels, reducing their response both to the constrictor effect of noradrenaline and to the dilator action of isoprenaline. Sedation, depression and dryness of the mouth occur, but its most important adverse effect is rebound hypertension associated with sudden termination of long-term therapy, the pharmacological mechanism of which is not yet known.

(e) Pargyline is a monoamine oxidase inhibitor. These drugs have paradoxical effects on blood pressure. Their hypertensive complications associated with the ingestion of tyramine-containing foodstuffs have already been discussed. Postural hypotension has been noted with several of these drugs, however, although the mechanism is unknown, and pargyline is the most consistent in its antihypertensive effects. However, it shares with the other drugs of this group the dangers of hypertensive crises, and also tends to promote fluid retention. It may unmask psychotic symptoms such as hallucinations and delusions.

(f) Sodium nitroprusside, given by carefully monitored intravenous infusion, has a direct dilator effect on vascular musculature independent of neural mechanisms. The effect is immediate, and ends as soon as the infusion is stopped. It is, therefore, of particular value in the management of very severe hypertension or its acute complications. It has few if any short-term toxic effects. Long-term effects are due to accumulation of thiocyanate to which nitroprusside is converted, and serum levels should, therefore, be measured at frequent intervals.

5-HYDROXYTRYPTAMINE

5-Hydroxytryptamine (5HT, serotonin) is widely distributed throughout the body, being concentrated in blood platelets and enterochromaffin cells of the gastrointestinal mucosa, which constitute the main storage sites of the body. It is synthesized from dietary tryptophan which is hydroxylated to 5-hydroxytryptophan (5HTP) and then decarboxylated to 5HT. Tumours of enterochromaffin cells, known as carcinoid tumours, produce excess of 5HT which contributes in part to the clinical picture of the condition.

5HT has a powerful vasoconstrictor effect which is direct and does not appear to involve nervous mechanisms. It also has strong contracting effects on various parts of the gastrointestinal tract. There is good evidence that 5HT is a transmitter in the central nervous systems (p. 61). Tissue levels are depleted by p-chlorophenylalanine which inhibits its synthesis, and reserpine which prevents its intracellular binding and thus leads to its destruction by monoamine oxidase.

5HT antagonists

Methysergide is a potent 5HT receptor blocking drug with partial agonist activity, which is used in the symptomatic treatment of the carcinoid syndrome and in the prophylaxis of migraine. A large number of adverse effects are associated with its use, including vomiting, abdominal cramps and diarrhoea. Severe peripheral vasoconstriction may also occur. More serious is the production of retroperitoneal fibrosis in patients treated for longer periods of time, and it is advisable to restrict its administration to periods of not more than 3 months.

Cyproheptadine antagonizes the action of 5HT and also of other pharmacological substances such as histamine and acetylcholine. It has other interesting actions such as stimulation of appetite leading to an increase in body weight, and is sometimes used clinically for this purpose. Drowsiness occurs commonly with its use, and its anticholinergic effects may lead to dryness of the mouth, and precipitation of glaucoma or urinary retention in predisposed patients.

6

Neuropharmacology

CNS TRANSMITTERS AND DRUG ACTION

Less is known about the transmitters in the brain and spinal cord than in the peripheral nervous system simply because of the complexity and inaccessibility of these structures. For this reason it is usually more difficult to explain the effects of a centrally-acting drug in terms of modification of transmitter action, although there are a growing number of examples where this is now possible, albeit a little tentatively in some cases. With other drugs it is possible to make little more than an inspired guess about their mode of action. If a chemical substance is to be considered as a putative transmitter in the central nervous system (CNS), it must satisfy several criteria: (a) it must occur naturally in the tissue, and be released by electrical stimulation, (b) enzymes for its synthesis and breakdown must be present, (c) local application or injection of the substance should mimic the action of the transmitter and (d) drugs which block synaptic transmission at this site should also block the effect of the locally-applied substance. Based on animal experiments, a number of substances satisfy these criteria either fully or in part.

Acetylcholine
This is found in considerable amounts in the tegmental pathways, cerebral cortex and basal ganglia, and is released from the cortex by electrical stimulation. Some cortical cells are excited by acetylcholine, while others are inhabited. Atropine can produce lack of concentration and memory, hallucinations and EEG alerting. Anticholinergic drugs used in Parkinsonism not infrequently precipitate toxic confusional states.

Noradrenaline
This is most abundant in nerve fibres in the hypothalamus, median eminence, olfactory bulb, limbic system, cranial nerve nuclei, and

the spinal cord. These nerve fibres arise almost exclusively from cell bodies in the lower brain stem, particularly in the pons, medulla and reticular formation. Drugs which modify noradrenergic transmission, such as monoamine oxidase inhibitors (MAOI), imipramine, amphetamine and reserpine, have marked effects on mood, motor activity, endocrine secretion from the pituitary, and body temperature. Circulating noradrenaline cannot cross the 'blood-brain barrier' (an anatomically ill-defined barrier which has the properties of a lipid membrane between the plasma and brain) but when injected into the cerebral ventricles it produces sedation.

Dopamine

In some nerve terminals the synthetic pathway producing catecholamines stops short at dopamine, and this substances appears to be the transmitter. Its importance in the neostriatum is established; degeneration of the nigro-striatal pathway, whose nerve terminals contain dopamine, leads to Parkinsonism. In addition, drugs which can block dopamine receptors, e.g. phenothiazines and butyrophenones, can produce Parkinsonism. Dopamine is involved in the inhibitory control of prolactin secretion from the anterior pituitary; drugs that block dopamine receptors cause hyperprolactinaemia.

5-Hydroxytryptamine

This substance is found in highest concentrations in the anterior part of the hypothalamus and amygdala. Fibres which contain 5HT arise mainly from cells in the midline raphe nuclei of the brain stem. Electrical stimulation of these nuclei produces alerting in experimental animals. On the other hand, a lesion destroying these fibres can produce insomnia. 5HT is synthesized from tryptophan as follows:

Tryptophan $\xrightarrow{\text{hydroxylation}}$ 5-hydroxytryptophan $\xrightarrow{\text{decarboxylation}}$ 5-hydroxy-

tryptamine.

Histamine

This can be found in synaptic vesicles in the hypothalamus, thalamus and cerebral cortex, although its possible role as a transmitter is undetermined.

Inhibitory amino acids
There are several of these substances, the most importance being
δ-aminobutyric acid (GABA) and glycine. The former is restricted
in its distribution to the central nervous system, and is present in
larger amounts than any of the other amino acids. It acts as a postsynaptic inhibitory transmitter in the cerebral and cerebellar cortex, whereas in the spinal cord it mediates presynaptic inhibition of
afferent pathways (Fig. 7). Glycine is found particularly in the
nerve terminals of spinal interneurones, and probably acts as a
postsynaptic inhibitory transmitter on motoneurones.

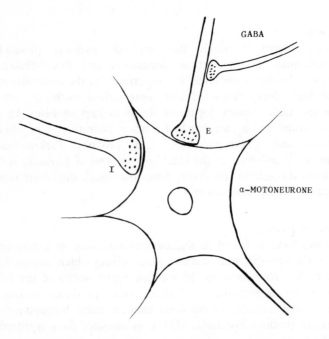

Fig. 7 Mechanisms of inhibition. The postsynaptic inhibitory terminal (I) synapses
directly with the α-motoneurone whereas the presynaptic inhibitory terminal
containing GABA synapses against the excitatory afferent terminal (E), depolarizing
it and reducing its output of transmitter.

Excitatory amino acids
The most widespread in their distribution are L-glutamic and
L-aspartic acids. They are released from the cerebral cortex when
the reticular formation is stimulated electrically. They excite many
different types of nerve cell, including cortical neurones and spinal
motoneurones.

Prostaglandins
Types E and F are widely distributed in the CNS and can produce a variety of effects when injected intravenously or applied directly to nerve cells, but a transmitter function has yet to be established for these substances.

Other putative neurotransmitters
Many other substances have been identified in the CNS which appear to satisfy some or all of the criteria demanded of a transmitter. These include substance P, vasoactive intestinal polypeptide, somatostatin, angiotensin and cholecystokinin, all of which are contained in afferent terminals in the spinal cord. In addition, the substantia gelatinosa contains enkephalins (see p. 113), neurotensin, neurophysin, oxytocin, glucagon, vasopressin, motilin and bombesin. A transmitter or modulator role is likely for at least some of these.

Modification of transmission
The central synapses which have been studied in greatest detail are those at which monoamines (noradrenaline, dopamine and 5HT) are the transmitters. The synthesis, release and fate of noradrenaline at the sympathetic postganglionic nerve terminal have been described in the last chapter. Central noradrenergic terminals are functionally similar to these. Figure 8 illustrates the sites at which some commonly used centrally-acting drugs modify transmission in these terminals. They can act in the following ways:

(a) *By modifying synthesis of monoamines* (Site I). The actions of α-methyl p-tyrosine and α-methyl dopa on sympathetic nerve terminals are described on pages 34 and 45. Both can affect catecholamine synthesis in the brain leading to sedation, and α-methyl dopa occasionally produces depression in patients treated with this drug for hypertension.

Levodopa is given to patients with Parkinson's disease with the object of building up the depleted levels of dopamine in the corpus striatum. Levodopa (L-dopa) is identical to the naturally occurring dopa which is produced in the synthetic pathway for catecholamines, and of the large dose which is taken orally by the patient a small percentage reaches the corpus striatum and is converted into dopamine in the nerve terminals. Unfortunately this conversion takes place at other catecholamine terminals in the central and sympathetic nervous systems, leading to frequent unwanted effects.

In the same way as levodopa builds up dopamine levels,

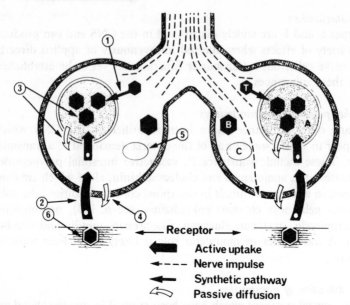

Fig. 8 Diagrammatic representation of a central adrenergic synapse showing possible sites of drug action. Right: A, granular pool of catecholamine; B, cytoplasmic pool of catecholamine; C, monoamine oxidase; T, precursors of catecholamines (tyrosine, etc.). Left: 1–6, see text.

L-tryptophan increases 5HT levels in central tryptaminergic terminals and this has been used as a supplementary treatment for depression.

(*b*) *By blocking re-uptake* (Site 2). Monoamines are taken up again into nerve terminals after they have been released by an impulse, and are transported back into the granular stores ready for subsequent release. A drug preventing this re-uptake will bring about an increase in the extraneuronal concentrations of noradrenaline and 5HT. This mechanism is thought to explain the therapeutic effects of the tricyclic antidepressants.

(*c*) *By modifying storage* (Site 3). Reserpine and a related compound, tetrabenazine, block the uptake of monoamines into the granular stores, as well as promoting their release from these stores. The granules thus become depleted and this impairs transmission. The released transmitter is deaminated by MAO before leaving the terminals, and no initial stimulant effect is seen. Depletion of noradrenaline, dopamine and 5HT results in sedation and reduced motor activity, and suicidal depression has occurred with higher doses of reserpine in hypertensive patients. The depletion of dopamine from the corpus striatum can lead to Parkinsonism, but is turned to therapeutic use in the treatment of dyskinesias.

(d) *By promoting release from the terminals* (Site 4). Some drugs, for example amphetamine, ephedrine and tyramine, are able to release monoamines from the nerve terminals in a physiologically-active form, mimicking transmission. They do not, however, deplete the granular stores to produce subsequent block.

(e) *By modifying breakdown* (Site 5). The most important enzyme concerned in the breakdown of monoamines is MAO, which is situated in the nerve terminals. Inhibition of this enzyme leads to accumulation of monoamines, which in turn brings about an elevation in mood.

(f) *By blocking postsynaptic receptors* (Site 6). Phenothiazine compounds have, to varying extents, both α-adrenoceptor and dopamine-receptor blocking activity, which is partly responsible for their effects on behaviour and motor activity. The butyrophenones have dopamine blocking effects, but only exhibit α-blocking actions in high doses. Both groups of compound frequently produce Parkinsonism when prescribed in high dosage. Although lysergic acid diethylamide (LSD) is a 5HT antagonist it is uncertain whether this accounts for the psychic changes which the drug can produce, for other analogues antagonize 5HT but do not induce psychoses.

(g) *By stimulating receptors* (Site 6). Bromocriptine probably produces its effects by direct stimulation of dopamine receptors in the CNS (p. 181).

DRUGS IN NEUROLOGY

Parkinsonism

Belladonna alkaloids were first used in the treatment of Parkinsonism just over 100 years ago, and anticholinergic drugs were the standard treatment until the 1960s, when further advances in therapy were stimulated by the observation that the concentration of dopamine in the corpus striatum of patients with idiopathic and postencephalitic Parkinsonism is reduced. Subsequently levodopa was administered to a few patients and encouraging results were obtained. This substance has emerged from innumerable clinical trials as the drug of choice in Parkinsonism.

The evidence for a regulatory mechanism in the striatum which is set by antagonistic effects of two transmitters, acetylcholine and dopamine, is now substantial, but the main points are as follows:

(a) Parkinsonism is alleviated by drugs which increase striatal dopamine or block the actions of acetylcholine.

(b) Drugs which deplete dopamine stores, e.g. reserpine, or block dopamine receptors, e.g. chlorpromazine, can induce or exacerbate Parkinsonism.

(c) Similarly, cholinomimetic or anticholinesterase drugs which penetrate into the brain, e.g. pilocarpine or physostigmine, worsen pre-existing disease.

(d) In experimental animals application of acetylcholine or carbachol to the caudate nucleus produces tremor and rigidity, which can be reversed by atropine or dopamine.

(e) Application of acetylcholine to single caudate neurones excites them, while dopamine usually inhibits them.

(f) The presence of high concentrations of acetylcholine, dopamine and the enzymes concerned in their synthesis and degradation have been demonstrated in the corpus striatum of animals and man.

The nerve terminals in the striatum which contain dopamine belong to a pathway from the substantia nigra, the nigro-striate pathway. Experimental lesions of these fibres in the monkey deplete striatal dopamine and produce contralateral hypokinesia and tremor. In patients with idiopathic and post-encephalitic Parkinsonism neuropathological studies have demonstrated a selective degeneration of this pathway, and examination of the CSF has shown low levels of homovanillic acid, the chief breakdown product of dopamine. The integrity of the cholinergic fibres terminating in the striatum appear to be unchanged, and normal concentrations of the enzymes concerned with the synthesis and breakdown of acetylcholine have been demonstrated.

All the evidence, therefore, points to a regulatory system in which acetylcholine is excitatory and dopamine is inhibitory to nerve cells concerned in extrapyramidal control, and that a disturbance of the balance of this system, in favour of acetylcholine, produces the clinical signs of Parkinsonism. A proposed scheme is illustrated in Figure 9. The treatment of the disease is directed to restoring the balance.

Anticholinergic drugs

A large number of naturally-occurring or synthetic anticholinergic drugs have been used in the treatment of Parkinsonism. Many of these have antihistamine properties in addition, but there is no evidence that this property is important. The more recent synthetic drugs do not seem to be superior to the more traditional compounds.

Only limited improvement is seen, rigidity responding best, tremor less well, and hypokinesia little, if at all. The aetiology of the disease does not influence the response, and neither does treatment modify the course of the disease. It may be necessary to try different combinations of drugs, gradually increasing to maximum dosage, before an adequate response is seen.

Benzhexol is one of the most satisfactory and popular of these drugs, and has moderate potency. Benztropine is a more powerful drug, and can be useful given parenterally in the treatment of phenothiazine-induced dyskinesias. Orphenadrine is a less powerful anticholinergic, produces fewer side-effects, and is said to have a euphoriant action which makes it the drug of choice in depressed patients. This may be explained by its ability to block reuptake of dopamine and other monoamines into nerve terminals. Other drugs include procyclidine, ethopropazine, methixine, cycrimine and biperiden.

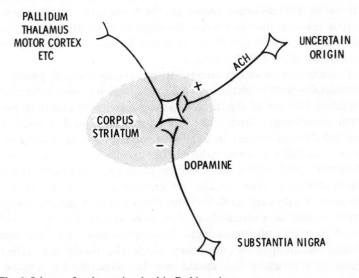

Fig. 9 Scheme of pathways involved in Parkinsonism.

The side-effects of these drugs are predictable from their pharmacological actions. Parasympathetic blockade produces dry mouth, blurred vision at near, constipation and hesitancy of micturition. Narrow angle glaucoma can be precipitated, and urinary retention can occur in males with prostatic hypertrophy. Confusion and hallucinations are seen in 20 to 30 per cent of patients receiving the more powerful anticholinergics, and should be treated by withdrawal of the drug, and, if necessary, administration of an anticholinesterase which gains access to the brain, e.g. physostigmine. However, sudden withdrawal of treatment in a patient deriving some therapeutic benefit can occasionally lead to a dramatic worsening of the clinical picture, out of all proportion to the improvement which the drug had been producing.

Levodopa

Dopamine does not penetrate into the brain, so striatal dopamine levels can be increased only by giving its precursor, L-dopa, which is converted to the transmitter by dopa decarboxylase. The racemic mixture, DL-dopa, caused frequent depression of the bone marrow.

The introduction of this drug represented a major advance in the treatment of a common and disabling disease. About one third of patients obtain very considerable benefit, the improvement occasionally being dramatic. Another third gain useful benefit, while the remainder are not helped or suffer disabling adverse effects. Idiopathic Parkinsonism shows the best response. Patients with postencephalitic disease tolerate levodopa poorly, often developing adverse effects with low doses. It is usually ineffective in patients with drug-induced Parkinsonism.

In contrast with anticholinergic drugs, levodopa usually produces considerable improvement in hypokinesia, which is one of the more disabling features of the disease. There is renewed ability to perform movements which have been lost for several years, and marked changes are seen in facial movements, walking, writing and speech. Rigidity is often reduced, but tremor is less consistently improved, and sometimes requires prolonged treatment before much change is seen. Oculogyric crises may be abolished, and drooling of saliva reduced. Previous treatment with anticholinergic drugs should be continued, as they have synergistic effects with levodopa, but phenothiazines, butyrophenones and reserpine should be stopped because they block the therapeutic effect. Pyridoxine (vitamin B6) should not be given during levodopa treatment because it is converted into pyridoxal phosphate which forms a coenzyme to dopa decarboxylase, enhancing the peripheral decarboxylation of the drug. Thus, less is available to enter the brain. Many vitamin mixtures and tonics contain pyridoxine, and patients should be warned of this. Levodopa should never be given to patients receiving a MAOI, for hypertensive crises can be provoked by doses as small as 50 mg.

Only a small fraction of the dose of levodopa reaches the corpus striatum and is converted into dopamine. The remainder is decarboxylated elsewhere, mainly peripherally. Carbidopa (as in Sinemet) and benserazide (as in Madopar) are decarboxylase inhibitors which cannot penetrate into the brain, and when given with levodopa block peripheral utilization without affecting central metabolism. This has the advantage of reducing the amount of levodopa which has to be administered to about a quarter, thereby reducing the number and size of tablets administered as well as lowering the incidence of gastrointestinal adverse effects. However, dyskinetic reactions may be more frequent because the brain levels of dopamine achieved are higher. Pyridoxine appears not to interfere with the therapeutic effects of combinations of levodopa and a peripheral decarboxylase inhibitor.

Levodopa is readily absorbed and produces a peak serum level at 1 to 2 hours, declining rapidly thereafter. Adverse effects, particularly gastrointestinal symptoms, coincide with the peak serum level, and are less if small frequent doses are given rather than larger infrequent ones.

Adverse effects of levodopa

Adverse effects are seen at some stage in the majority of patients treated with the drug. They include:

(a) *Gastrointestinal symptoms.* Anorexia, nausea and vomiting are the commonest problems while the dose is being increased. Slowing the rate of increase helps. These effects are probably central in origin, but can be reduced by taking the drug immediately after food, which delays absorption. Once the dose is stabilized these symptoms almost always settle.

(b) *Postural hypotension.* The mechanism of this effect is uncertain. It has been suggested that dopamine might be acting as a false transmitter at sympathetic nerve terminals, but recent work presents evidence for a central site of action.

(c) *Dyskinesia.* Involuntary movements are very common at higher dose levels, although in patients with postencephalitic Parkinsonism they may appear early in treatment. They first appear in the tongue and facial muscles, and lip-smacking movements are often the first sign. The movements may spread to the neck, trunk and limbs. They often appear several weeks after the patient has reached a stable dose level. When this occurs a reduction in the dose is necessary.

(d) *Psychiatric disturbances.* These occur in about 15 per cent of patients, and include anxiety, restlessness, depression, confusion and delusions. Occasionally frank psychosis may occur. These disturbances make it necessary to abandon treatment and attempts at continuing at a lower dose or restarting treatment later usually provoke further reactions. Patients with a history of psychiatric disturbance should not be considered for levodopa therapy.

(e) *Other adverse effects.* Occasionally, transient exacerbation of hypokinesia, so called 'on-off attacks', occur, particularly in patients treated with high doses of the drug. Cardiac dysrhythmias and angina have been reported and patients with a history of heart disease should be admitted to hospital for institution of therapy. A positive Coombs' test occurs rarely. Tachypnoea and fine tremor are occasionally seen.

Amantadine

This was developed as an antiviral drug in influenza, but its anti-Parkinsonian effect was noticed in a clinical trial. Its mode of action is uncertain, but it may act in an amphetamine-like manner, releasing catecholamines from nerve terminals. The clinical improvement induced by amantadine is much less than that produced by levodopa, but it is an easier drug to manage and the side-effects are fewer. Improvement is seen in all three major features, hypokinesia, rigidity and tremor. Drug-induced Parkinsonism does not respond.

The adverse effects of amantadine are dry mouth, defective near vision, constipation, confusion and hallucinations. A bluish-red skin discolouration, livideo reticularis, occurs in most patients, and ankle oedema is common.

Other drugs

Amphetamine has a beneficial effect in Parkinsonism, probably by releasing dopamine from nerve endings or preventing reuptake of released dopamine into the terminals. The therapeutic effect, however, is mild and risks of habituation preclude its use. Bromocriptine, a directly acting dopamine agonist, is probably no more effective than levodopa plus a decarboxylase inhibitor, and may be more toxic. It is used also in treating galactorrhoea and acromegaly (p. 181).

Dyskinesia

Disturbance of extrapyramidal function can produce a number of syndromes in which involuntary movements predominate. The effectiveness of reserpine in Huntington's chorea was noted some years ago, but the drug produced many side-effects, particularly depression. Tetrabenazine is a drug with similar pharmacological actions, and trials have shown it to be effective in Huntington's chorea, other choreiform syndromes, dystonia and hemiballismus. Therapy is easier to manage, as it produces its effects quickly, and has a short duration of action compared with reserpine. These drugs are presumably producing their effects in these patients by depleting monoamines, and support is given to this suggested mode of action by the observation that subjects dying with Huntington's chorea have an increase in dopamine concentration in the corpus striatum and pars compacta of the substantia nigra, as well as in the nucleus accumbens.

Phenothiazines can also reduce abnormal movements, presumably by virtue of their blocking effects at central monoaminergic receptors. Thiopropazate, a piperazine derivative, seems to be of particular value in this respect.

Drug-induced extrapyramidal syndromes

The relationship between central catecholamine metabolism and extrapyramidal syndromes is a complex one. Depletion of the stores in nerve terminals with reserpine produces Parkinsonism, while increasing the concentration of catecholamines with levodopa leads to dyskinesia. Between these two extremes is a spectrum of disorders, most of which can be produced at various times by the phenothiazines. Acute dystonic reactions tend to occur in young patients, akathisia (motor restlessness) and tasikinesia (an inability to remain seated) in the middle aged, while Parkinsonism is the most common syndrome in the elderly. These reactions are usually reversible on stopping the offending drug. In contrast, irreversible dyskinesias can be produced by phenothiazines, and occur much more frequently than is generally realized, possibly in up to 25 per cent of institutionalized patients. The complexity of these reactions is further illustrated by the fact the phenothiazines which produce dyskinesias in some patients can be useful for treating these conditions in others.

Drug-induced Parkinsonism is little improved by levodopa or amantadine. Where withdrawal of the offending drug is not possible, as is usually the case in schizophrenia, addition of an anticholinergic drug is helpful.

Levodopa-induced dyskinesia is almost invariably reversible, unlike its phenothiazine counterpart. Although it can be effectively treated with tetrabenazine or thiopropazate, these drugs also reverse the anti-Parkinsonian action, so it is more rational to reduce the dose of levodopa.

Epilepsy

Ideas on the classification of the epilepsies have changed in recent years, and with this change drug treatment has become more rational. The high incidence of partial (focal) epilepsy, especially temporal lobe epilepsy, has been recognized, and, in addition, the distinction between absence (petit mal) attacks and minor temporal lobe seizures has been more clearly defined, largely as a result of improved EEG techniques. Tonic-clonic (grand mal) and partial seizures are treated primarily with hydantoins, carbamazepine and barbiturates, while absence seizures respond to treatment with suc- cinimides and sodium valproate. Sometimes absences and tonic clonic seizures coexist, demanding combined therapy.

Hydantoins

These include phenytoin (diphenylhydantoin), ethotoin and methoin. The first of these is the most widely used drug in major epilepsy. It is hydroxylated in the liver by an enzyme system which

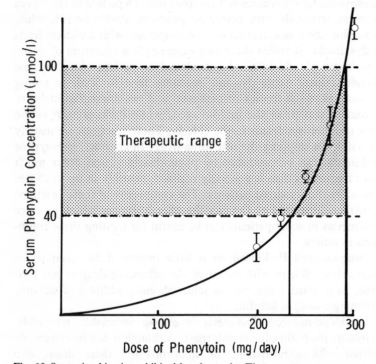

Fig. 10 Saturation kinetics exhibited by phenytoin. The measurements were obtained from one patient on several maintenance doses of phenytoin, and show a curvilinear relationship with a small dose range compatible with a therapeutic serum concentration.

is saturable, and in some patients up to 20 days may be required for the serum level to stabilize after changing the dose. The rate of metabolism of the drug varies greatly between patients, and one may be intoxicated by a dose which is therapeutically ineffective in another. Because of this it is necessary to increase the dose gradually until fit control is achieved or until signs of intoxication occur. The triad of signs which indicate overdosage are nystagmus, ataxia, and dysarthria, signs of deranged cerebellar and brain stem function. If these signs are ignored permanent damage can result. Because of these uncertainties estimation of the serum level of the drug is invaluable. The aim is to produce a serum level of up to 100 μmol/1 (25 μg/ml). The relationship between dose and serum level is a non-linear one, typical of saturation kinetics, and therefore increments in dose should become progressively smaller as the therapeutic range is reached (Fig. 10). Once-daily dosage gives stable control in adults, although twice-daily administration is preferable in children, who metabolize drugs more quickly.

Although phenytoin lacks the sedative property of phenobarbitone, it produces a greater variety of adverse reactions (see below). Inevitably there are differences of opinion as to which is preferable.

Phenytoin is effective in suppressing tonic-clonic seizures, or the spread of a focal fit to a generalized one, but it is less valuable in suppressing the focus itself, including a temporal lobe focus. It is of no value in absence seizures unless tonic-clonic attacks coexist. Phenytoin has diverse pharmacological actions, including a direct depressant effect on the excitable membrane, enhancement of potassium transport into nerve cells, and effects on the metabolism of GABA. Which, if any, accounts for its anticonvulsant effect is not known. It also has a membrane stabilizing effect on the myocardium, and is a useful antidysrhythmic drug (p. 131).

Methoin is more toxic than phenytoin, particularly on the bone marrow. Ethotoin is much less effective, although it is also less toxic.

Carbamazepine

Although related to the tricyclic antidepressants, carbamazepine is an effective anticonvulsant in tonic-clonic and partial seizures. It is probably as effective as phenytoin and phenobarbitone in tonic-clonic fits and may be superior to these two in partial epilepsies, in which it is regarded as a drug of first choice by some authorities. It is to be preferred to barbiturates because it is less sedative, although dizziness is a common adverse effect. A psychotropic action has been claimed but poorly substantiated, and may simply be an artefact produced by changing from sedative barbiturate drugs to a compound which is less toxic on the central nervous system.

Initially, carbamazepine acquired the reputation of being toxic on the bone marrow. Further experience has shown that, although rare cases of fatal agranulocytosis have been reported, the drug is remarkably safe in the epileptic patient. Bone marrow toxicity appears to be more common when the drug is used in trigeminal neuralgia, perhaps because of the greater age of patients with this condition.

Carbamazepine has a shorter serum half-life than phenytoin, particularly in patients receiving combination therapy (its metabolism is inducible) and therefore it needs to be given two or three times daily. It is a potent liver enzyme inducing drug itself, and can therefore induce its own metabolism as well as that of other drugs. Its major metabolite is an epoxide, which also possesses antiepileptic activity, although somewhat less than the parent compound.

Barbiturates

The introduction in 1912 of phenobarbitone for the treatment of grand mal epilepsy provided a potent anticonvulsant which has been one of the mainstays of treatment ever since. Only the long-acting barbiturates, e.g. barbitone, phenobarbitone and methyl-phenobarbitone, have useful anticonvulsant properties for oral treatment of chronic epilepsy. Some of the short-acting compounds actually have convulsant properties, and are used for activating epileptic foci in diagnostic electroencephalography, although they can, paradoxically, be of value in the treatment of status (see below). Phenobarbitone is the most widely used barbiturate. Because it is metabolized only slowly in the liver, and only about 30 per cent is excreted unchanged in the urine, it is cumulative and takes about 30 days to reach a constant serum level. Hasty changes of treatment should not, therefore, be made, and 3 months or more may be required to assess the value of the drug adequately in any one patient. The drug should be given in one dose at night.

Sedation is one of the chief drawbacks of phenobarbitone, and often limits the dose. It is worse during the period when the dose is being built up, but tends to settle when a steady dose is arrived at. This is the result of tolerance, and withdrawal symptoms can occur after stopping the drug. These withdrawal symptoms include epileptic fits, and therefore reductions in dose should be made very gradually. Sudden withdrawal of phenobarbitone can precipitate status epilepticus. Phenobarbitone is poorly tolerated in children, causing impairment of learning capacity, irritability and disturbances of behaviour. If it is necessary to give a drug for tonic-clonic seizures to a child it is better to choose carbamazepine or sodium valproate.

These adverse effects make phenobarbitone no longer a drug of first choice in tonic-clonic and partial seizures. It should be used only when phenytoin or carbamazepine have been ineffective. The mode of action of the anticonvulsant barbiturates is uncertain, although it may be no more than the result of a generalized depressant effect on nerve cell membranes or presynaptic terminals.

Primidone is structurally closely related to the barbiturates and is, in fact, converted partly into phenobarbitone by liver enzymes. For this reason combinations of phenobarbitone and primidone should be avoided if at all possible, for they have additive sedative effects. Some patients are intolerant of primidone, and an initial test dose of half a tablet is advisable. Blood dyscrasias are more common with this drug than with phenobarbitone.

Sodium valproate

This compound is structurally very different from any other antiepileptic drug, being a simple two chain fatty acid. It inhabits enzymes which are responsible for GABA metabolism in the brain, which may partly account for its antiepileptic effects. It has a broad spectrum of action, and it is a drug of first choice in both absence and myoclonic seizures. It has an advantage over ethosuximide for these types of seizures in that it is also active against co-existing tonic-clonic fits. In partial seizures it is less impressive and will probably not replace the more established drugs.

It is relatively free from adverse effects, but will potentiate the sedative effects of phenobarbitone and primidone by inhibiting their metabolism. Increased appetite and reversible hair loss have been described. Hepatotoxicity has been reported, rarely fatal. It has a short half-life, but, paradoxically, it has a long duration of action (a 'hit-and-run' type of action) and once-daily dosage appears to be satisfactory.

Succinimides

These compounds are used for the treatment of absences and myoclonic seizures. In tonic-clonic and partial seizures they are ineffective. Ethosuximide is most commonly used, but methsuximide is an alternative. These drugs can be combined with any of those for major epilepsy when both types of fit coexist but single drug treatment wtih sodium valproate is preferable. Ethosuximide has a long serum half-life, and once daily dosage is satisfactory.

Toxic effects include nausea and vomiting, dizziness and drowsiness, and leucopenia.

Oxazolidinediones

Paramethadione and trimethadione (troxidone) were the predecessors to the succinimides. They are now infrequently used because they are less effective than the succinimides and are more toxic. Adverse effects include glare phenomenon and photobia, skin rashes, blood dyscrasias and hepatic and renal damage.

Benzodiazepines

The benzodiazepine drugs are widely used for treating status epilepticus (see below) although their long-term oral use in epilepsy has been disappointing, possibly because central tolerance has occurred and the dose has not been increased adequately to compensate for this. The most potent anticonvulsant benzodiazepine, clonazepam, is effective in absences and myoclonic seizures, but is very sedative. Sodium valproate should always be tried first. Nitrazepam has been widely used in massive infantile spasms (salaam spasms, hypsarrhythmia), although the evidence for its effectiveness is not satisfactory. ACTH and oral steroids are of value in this condition.

Other anticonvulsants

Sulthiame has been widely used for treating major epilepsy. Although it has shown anticonvulsant activity in animals, it probably works in man mainly by inhibiting the metabolism of other drugs for major epilepsy which are given concurrently. It is wiser simply to increase the dose of these latter drugs if fits remain uncontrolled. Sulthiame can cause parasthesiae and hyperpnoea. Beclamide, a drug which is said to have stimulant rather than sedative properties, is only a weak anticonvulsant and is little used. Acetazolamide, the carbonic anhydrase inhibitor and diuretic, has been used in petit mal absences, but its effect is not impressive.

Adverse effects of long-term anticonvulsant therapy

It is sometimes necessary to treat a patient simultaneously with two or even three drugs in order to control major fits. Sedation from the barbiturates and cerebellar disturbance by the hydantoins are frequently dose limiting. But apart from these signs of intoxication, a number of abnormalities are produced by chronic disturbance of many metabolic pathways which results from ingestion of large amounts of these drugs for many years. The more important of these effects are:

(a) *Gum hypertrophy*. This odd effect is produced almost exclusively by the hydantoins, but the reason is unknown. On the whole it is dose related, but some patients are much more sensitive to this effect than others. It can be so gross as to overgrow the teeth and impair occlusion, leading in turn to dental sepsis and halitosis. It is unsightly and, naturally enough, intolerable to young ladies. It does not occur in the edentulous.

(b) *Acne, greasy skin and hirsutes*. Again, these effects are unexplained, but are disfiguring.

(c) *Lymphadenopathy, simulating Hodgkin's disease*. This is a benign condition and subsides on withdrawal of the offending drug, usually a hydantoin.

(d) *Systemic lupus erythematosus*. Like procainamide, the anticonvulsants can occasionally cause this condition.

(e) *Liver enzyme induction*. Stimulation of certain enzyme systems by these potent inducing drugs can increase the rate of metabolism of themselves and other drugs or of endogenous compounds.

(f) *Folate deficiency*. Up to 50 per cent of patients have a low serum folate level, and many of these have a true tissue deficiency. Despite this, megaloblastic anaemia occurs only rarely, and there is no adequate evidence that this disturbance has any other adverse consequences. It is therefore unnecessary to give folic acid supplements unless macrocytic changes occur. The mechanism of the effect is uncertain.

(g) *Osteomalacia*. Biochemical changes of osteomalacia, and sometimes frank bone disease, are seen, probably as a result of modified vitamin D metabolism in the liver.

(h) *Foetal abnormalities*. The incidence of malformations, especially of hare lip and cleft palate, is greater than average in the babies of epileptic mothers and may be partly due to drug therapy. In addition, a bleeding tendency may be present at birth because the production of clotting factors in the neonate is disturbed.

Drugs for status epilepticus

Fits are potentially damaging to the brain. This applies particularly to status in childhood, which can lead to permanent temporal lobe damage, and this can in turn result in temporal lobe epilepsy. Status is therefore an emergency and should be terminated as quickly as possible. Diazepam given intravenously is regarded as the drug of choice. Sometimes its effect is only transient, and it may have to be given in repeated doses. Infusion over long periods should be avoided, however, because prolonged coma can result from accumulation of N-desmethyldiazepam, which is only slowly eliminated (p. 103). Diazepam causes significant respiratory depression and hypotension only when other drugs, e.g. phenobarbitone, have been given parenterally before it. Clonazepam may be even more effective than diazepam. Intravenous phenytoin is an alternative, given as a loading dose of 1000 mg (assuming the patient has not been on chronic phenytoin therapy) followed by a daily maintenance dose. Intramuscularly, phenytoin is highly irritant and badly absorbed. Phenobarbitone is unsatisfactory in status because it penetrates the blood-brain barrier only slowly. If diazepam is used initially to stop the acute episode, phenytoin or phenobarbitone should subsequently be administered parenterally to prevent recurrence. Thiopentone, or some other short-acting barbiturate, given as an initial intravenous injection may be effective, but infusion should be avoided because the elimination half-life of the drug is long (unlike the distribution half life which determines the duration of unconsciousness after a single dose) and, like diazepam, prolonged coma can result. Paraldehyde given intramuscularly, or slowly intravenously after dilution, is still used by some. It is relatively safe, although it has a number of disadvantages. Chlormethiazole given by infusion is effective, but not widely used.

Occasionally status may be resistant to one or several of the above drugs. It may then be necessary to anaesthetise and curarize the patient and maintain breathing by intermittent positive pressure ventilation through a tracheostomy tube.

Drugs which can cause fits
It is important to bear in mind the potential convulsant action of some drugs, for they should not, if possible, be given to epileptic patients, and they may occasionally precipitate a fit in a patient who has never previously had one. Drugs possessing this action include the phenothiazines, tricyclic antidepressants, aminophylline and many antihistamines. Abrupt withdrawal of barbiturates or benzodiazepines can also precipitate fits. Drugs given intrathecally, especially penicillin and antimitotic drugs readily produce fits. Needless to say, an epileptic should not be given analeptic drugs.

Narcolepsy
This is a rare condition which includes an uncontrollable desire to sleep, hypnogogic hallucinations, and sleep paralysis.

Amphetamine is the best treatment but the tricyclic antidepressants, particularly clomipramine, are effective when cataplexy is prominent.

Migraine

The aetiology of migraine is disputed. Most theories have centred around a vascular origin for the pain, resulting from a dilatation of cranial vessels. Several chemical theories have been put forward to explain this dilatation, including a change in levels of circulating histamine, acetylcholine, 5HT and, most recently, prostaglandins. An alternative explanation is that migraine arises in the brain stem as a paroxysmal sympathetic discharge. The demonstration of a reduced venous 5HT level in migraine, and the prophylactic value of methysergide, a potent 5HT antagonist, have lent support to the view that this monoamine is involved in the genesis of migraine attacks, but the results of the 5HT measurements require corroboration. A defect in tyramine metabolism has been suggested, and would explain the association between various foods and migraine attacks in some patients. The high incidence of non-specific EEG abnormalities have led some to postulate a cerebral cause for the attacks, and phenytoin has been claimed to be of value in treatment. Because of these uncertainties about the aetiology of the disease, there is no logical treatment. Nausea and gastric stasis may occur early in a migraine attack, reducing the absorption of analgesic drugs given by the oral route. Metoclopramide, administered parenterally or rectally, may increase the rate of gastric emptying and so improve the absorption of analgesic drugs from the gastrointestinal tract. Traditional antiemetics such as cyclizine or prochlorperazine are less useful because their anticholinergic effects may adversely affect gastrointestinal motility.

Mild analgesics

These should be tried first, for they benefit a substantial proportion of patients, and have fewer side-effects. Aspirin and paracetamol are satisfactory. Soluble and effervescent preparations act more quickly.

Ergotamine tartrate

This is frequently of value in classical migraine when taken at the first warning of an attack. It is valueless if it is taken when the attack is established. In addition to its α-adrenolytic action, ergotamine has a direct constrictor effect on vascular smooth muscle, reversing the dilatation of cranial vessels.

The drug can be given in a variety of ways and forms. Intramuscular injection is probably the most satisfactory, but is often impractical. Inhalation by aerosol (Medihaler—ergotamine) is rapidly effective. The drug is absorbed from the buccal mucous membrane, and sublingual tablets (Lingraine) or tablets for chewing (Cafergot-Q) are useful. Oral administration is the most popular, although the drug is absorbed less rapidly. Absorption appears to be increased by addition of caffeine, which a number of proprietary preparations contain. The content of ergotamine varies from 1 to 2 mg, but no more than 12 mg should be taken in a week. Overdosage can cause peripheral vasoconstriction (St. Anthony's fire), gangrene of the extremities and headaches which may mimic the migraine syndrome which is being treated. Ergot-containing drugs should be avoided in pregnancy and cardiovascular disease. They should not be used for prophylaxis in migraine, although in cluster headaches it may be helpful.

Dihydroergotamine less frequently produces side-effects, but is probably also less effective. Its use in prophylaxis is acceptable.

Prophylactic drugs

Propranol is often helpful in reducing the frequency of migraine attacks. It is of interest in this respect that it has serotonin antagonist effects in addition to its β-blocking activity. It should not be given with ergotamine because they both increase peripheral resistance.

Pizotifen is structurally similar to cyproheptadine and the tricyclic antidepressants, and is a serotonin antagonist. It is often effective in prophylaxis but drowsiness and weight gain are common.

Another serotonin antagonist, methysergide is an effective drug in preventing attacks, but its chief disadvantage is the frequency, and occasional severity, of adverse effects. Nausea, drowsiness and unsteadiness are common, and peripheral vasoconstriction occurs, producing numbness, parasthesiae and muscle cramps. Perceptual changes and hallucinations have been seen. But the most serious complication is retroperitoneal fibrosis, leading to hydronephrosis. Fibrosis in pleural and pericardial cavities has occurred.

Clonidine (p. 58) reduces the responsiveness of peripheral vessels to both dilator and constrictor effects of catecholamines, which may account for its effectiveness as a prophylactic drug in migraine. It is given in much smaller doses than for hypertension, and with these doses adverse effects are few. It has not, however, been used for long enough to be fully evaluated.

Trigeminal neuralgia

Injection of alcohol or phenol into the gasserian ganglion, as was once the standard treatment for trigeminal neuralgia, has now been made obsolete by an effective drug, carbamazepine, which was introduced initially for epilepsy (p. 73). Whether trigeminal neuralgia is caused by an 'epileptiform' discharge somewhere along the trigeminal sensory pathway is disputed. Other anticonvulsant drugs, e.g. phenytoin, have also been used, but are less effective.

Bell's palsy

Although the cause of this condition is not known, there is evidence that ACTH and steroids reduce the incidence, and lessen the severity, of denervation when given in high dosage as soon after the onset of symptoms as possible. Steroids may be preferable to ACTH.

Spasticity

In spasticity there is an increase in the excitability either of spinal α-motoneurones or of fusimotor neurones; sometimes both are hyperactive. This is caused by an imbalance of descending excitatory and inhibitory tone resulting from a lesion of the corticospinal pathway, although the nature of the change in transmitter action is unknown. However, this abnormal state of affairs can be reversed either by reducing descending facilitation from the brain stem, or by a direct action on synaptic transmission in the spinal cord. Several tranquillizers have actions at both levels, but the relative importance of these mechanisms in producing the muscle relaxant effect of these drugs is uncertain. None of them is entirely satisfactory, for sedation often becomes a problem before much relief from spasticity has been achieved.

Diazepam (p. 103) is one of the more effective compounds for treating spasticity, and probably works mainly by facilitating GABA transmission in the spinal cord. GABA is known to act as a transmitter mediating presynaptic inhibition (Fig. 7), and benzodiazepines are thought to act on specific benzodiazepine receptors which enhance the postsynaptic affects of GABA. Diazepam is the most active of the benzodiazepines on muscle tone. Occasionally, extensor hypotonus can occur, making walking so difficult that treatment has to be discontinued.

Baclofen is a new addition to the range of antispasticity drugs, and structurally is very different. Although it is a derivative of GABA, the transmitter concerned in presynaptic inhibition in the spinal cord, it probably acts as a general neuronal depressant in the spinal cord rather than by mimicking GABA. It is a drug of first choice in spasticity, but frequently produces nausea, dizziness and hypotension.

Dantrolene is a hydantoin which impairs excitation contraction coupling in skeletal muscle, and appears to be useful in spasticity. It commonly causes muscle weakness, light headedness and diarrhoea.

A number of miscellaneous drugs, including methocarbamol, chlormezanone and styramate are of little practical value although they continue to be marketed for muscle spasm associated with minor sprains and injuries. Quinine is used for relieving nocturnal leg cramps.

Neuromuscular junction

Neuromuscular blocking drugs

The neuromuscular junction can be blocked in one of two ways, (a) by competitive inhibition, whereby the blocking drug antagonizes acetylcholine in proportion to its concentration at the receptor site, and (b) by depolarization of the end plate beyond the threshold required to generate an action potential in the muscle fibre. As the triggering threshold is passed an action potential may be produced, accounting for the initial muscle twitching which depolarizing drugs produce. This often causes subsequent aching in the muscles, no doubt resulting from slight damage produced by incoordinated contractions. The competitive antagonists do not have this effect, and they can prevent the twitching from depolarizing drugs when given in small dosage just before administration of the depolarizer. In addition to depolarization, the depolarizing drugs appear to produce a degree of desensitization of the receptors to acetylcholine, and this may in part account for their blocking action. Competitive blockade can be reversed by an anti-cholinesterase drug, which prevents breakdown of the transmitter and leads to its accumulation at the receptor site, changing the balance of concentrations in favour of acetycholine. Anti-cholinesterases deepen, rather than reverse, a depolarizing block, for accumulation of acetylcholine produces further depolarization. In fact, anticholinesterases in sufficient doses can themselves produce muscle fasciculation and depolarizing block.

Tubocurarine and gallamine are the two commonly used competitive drugs. Up to 3 minutes is required for maximum effect after injection. The action of gallamine lasts for 20 to 30 minutes, while tubocurarine has a slightly longer action. Gallamine can cause tachycardia from vagal inhibition, and tubocurarine produces slight hypotension from ganglionic blockade, and occasional histamine release.

Suxamethonium (succinyl choline) is the only useful depolarizing drug. It acts in 1 minute and its effects last for up to 5 minutes making it suitable for short anaesthetic procedures such as ECT. It has slight muscarinic effects, causing bradycardia from vagal stimulation. It should not be mixed with thiopentone in a syringe, for the alkalinity of the latter drug causes hydrolysis of suxamethonium. Plasma cholinesterase hydrolyses the drug to succinyl monocholine and finally succinic acid and choline, and enzyme variants can occasionally result in prolonged paralysis and apnoea. A pair of non-dominant autosomal genes determines the type of enzyme. Heterozygotes (3 per cent of the population) may have slightly delayed recovery, while homozygotes for the atypical gene (0·03 per cent) may take many hours to regain spontaneous breathing. Enzyme variants can be detected by measuring the degree to which the local anaesthetic, dibucaine, inhibits the enzyme.

Neuromuscular blocking drugs can be potentiated by aminoglycoside antibiotics, particularly neomycin, kanamycin and streptomycin, and by chlorpromazine and some general anaesthetic agents. Long-acting anticholinesterases used in the prophylactic treatment of glaucoma, can cause resistance to competitive antagonists. Patients with latent or overt myasthenia are particularly sensitive to neuromuscular blockade, and this has occasionally been used as a diagnostic test, but one which requires ventilation apparatus close to hand.

Anticholinesterases

These compounds impede the action of cholinesterase in one of two ways, either (1) by possessing a kationic group, usually a quaternary ammonium, which has affinity for the anionic site of the enzyme, thus preventing the union of enzyme and substrate, or (2) by acting as a false substrate, but one which forms an intermediate compound which can only by hydrolyzed slowly ('reversible') or not at all ('irreversible'). Edrophonium has the first type of action, while all the other commonly used drugs act as false substrates. Physostigmine, neostigmine and pyridostigmine form intermediate compounds which are hydrolyzed in a matter of hours, and the enzyme is released again for combination with acetyl choline, but the organophosphorus compounds produce stable intermediates, and new cholinesterase has to be synthesized, which may take up to several weeks to be complete.

Anticholinesterases have several clinical uses.

(a) Reversal of competitive neuromuscular blockade following surgery. Neostigmine remains the most useful drug for this purpose.

(b) Diagnosis of myasthenia gravis, or differential diagnosis between cholinergic crisis and myasthenic weakness (see below).

(c) Treatment of myasthenia gravis (see below).

(d) Treatment of paralytic ileus, bladder atony or supraventricular tachycardia. A drug with marked muscarinic effects, such as neostigmine, is required for this purpose.

(e) Treatment of glaucoma. Eye drops containing physostigmine, neostigmine or an organophosphorous compound can be used to keep the pupil constricted in narrow angle glaucoma.

Edrophonium has predominantly nicotinic effects, some of which are the result of direct stimulation of receptors in addition to its anticholinesterase activity, and it can cause muscle fasciculation in small doses or a depolarization block in larger doses. Its effects last for 10 minutes. Neostigmine has a longer duration of action, producing a useful effect for up to 4 hours or more. Its marked muscarinic effects are a disadvantage when the drug is being used for its neuromuscular actions, and often require addition of atropine or a similar drug to block muscarinic receptors. This is especially so when it is given to patients with myasthenia, when intestinal colic is frequently produced. Physostigmine is now obsolete clinically, except for its use in glaucoma. Pyridostigmine is a longer-acting preparation than neostigmine, and is used in treating myasthenia. Ambenonium, a quaternary ammonium compound, has an even longer duration of action, and may be cumulative when given regularly.

The organophosphorus compounds, e.g. dyflos, echothiophate and tetraethylpyrophosphate, have been developed primarily as insecticides or 'nerve gases', but are of value for long-term treatment of glaucoma, for which they are instilled into the eye in an oily vehicle once every few days. Unfortunately, they may cause anterior lens opacities and other ocular effects, and may be sufficiently absorbed systemically to produce resistance to competitive neuromuscular blockade, or even frank muscarinic effects. Poisoning with these compounds can be a serious matter, but the development of cholinesterase reactivators has provided an effective treatment. These drugs, e.g. pralidoxime (P2S), combine with the phosphorylated enzyme but have a greater affinity for the organophosphorus moiety, breaking its linkage with the enzyme. The reactivator must be given as soon as possible, certainly within a few hours, to be effective, for a chemical change in the organophosphorus–enzyme complex slowly takes place and a much more stable compound results.

Myasthenia gravis

In myasthenia gravis there is an impairment of transmission at the neuromuscular junction, the cause of which is still not clear. Failure of acetylcholine synthesis or release, or insensitivity of the end plate receptors to acetylcholine, possibly as a result of a circulating curare-like or antineuronal substance, have all been considered. Treatment is aimed at increasing the concentration of free acetylocholine at the junction, by inhibiting cholinesterase with anticholinesterase drugs, and this overcomes the deficient transmission. However, in excess, anticholinesterases can produce muscle fasciculation and depolarization block, and for each patient there is an optimum dose which produces maximum benefit without causing block, the so-called 'cholinergic crisis'. A patient with severe myasthenia usually has a lower plateau of response, and it is these patients in whom overdosage is most likely to occur. Sometimes it is impossible to distinguish between a worsening myasthenic state and a cholinergic crisis without resorting to a pharmacological test. Here the short duration of action of edrophonium is invaluable. An intravenous injection of 2 mg will produce prompt improvement when myasthenic weakness is the main problem, but will briefly worsen neuromuscular transmission in a cholinergic crisis. This test is also useful in the diagnosis of myasthenia gravis, which is the only form of muscle weakness which will respond to an anticholinesterase.

For regular maintenance therapy these drugs are given orally. Neostigmine is still the mainstay of treatment, although some consider that its duration of action is too short, so that the effect wears off overnight leaving the patient weak on awakening. When this occurs, pyridostigmine should be chosen for its longer duration of action. It may, in addition, produce fewer unwanted muscarinic effects. Ambenonium has an even longer action, but it seems to possess no advantage over pyridostigmine and yet produces a greater risk of accumulation and overdosage.

Severe intoxication with anticholinesterase drugs, causing embarrassed breathing and swallowing, can be treated with an intravenous oxime cholinesterase reactivator, but this is seldom necessary. Temporary withdrawal of the drug is all that need be done in most cases. Unwanted muscarinic effects are frequently troublesome, particularly after the first dose of the day, but can be prevented by addition of atropine or a similar muscarinic blocking drug which may require parenteral administration because of gastro-intestinal hurry.

Ephedrine has a slight stimulant effect at the neuromuscular junction, probably by increasing transmitter release (Orbelli phenomenon). It has long been used as adjuvant therapy, but its value is limited, and it can produce insomnia if taken too late in the day.

ACTH and steroids have recently been tried in patients who derive little benefit from conventional therapy. Long-term improvement has been reported, but at the expense of an initial deterioration which makes it imperative that treatment is started where there is access to an intensive-care unit.

In view of the important role of potassium ions in synaptic transmission oral potassium chloride has been tried, but with little success. Spironolactone, the potassium-retaining aldosterone antagonist, has been claimed to be of value but this is not generally accepted. There is a place for its use, however, when steroids are being given in large doses, for their mineralocorticoid effects cause potassium loss.

Several drugs are capable of causing or precipitating a myasthenic state in some patients. These include the aminoglycoside antibiotics streptomycin, neomycin and kanamycin, and phenytoin and phenothiazines.

ANTI-EMETICS

Central vomiting can be induced by stimulation either of the emetic centre in the brain stem, or of the chemoreceptor trigger zone (CTZ) situated in the floor of the fourth ventricle. Various centrally-acting emetic drugs act by stimulating the CTZ, but they will cause vomiting only when the emetic centre is intact, for it is the final common pathway for all emetic stimuli. Two classes of compound are useful anti-emetics, phenothiazines and anticholinergic drugs. The former block emetic stimuli acting through the CTZ whereas the latter act directly on the emetic centre. Some antihistamines also have effective anti-emetic properties, but these are probably accounted for by the marked anticholinergic actions of these compounds. Phenothiazines have atropine-like actions also, and they probably act on the emetic centre in addition to their effect on the CTZ. Figure 11 summarizes the various stimuli which can evoke central vomiting.

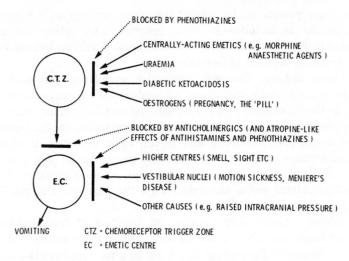

Fig. 11 Stimuli which can produce central vomiting, and their blockade by antiemetic drugs.

Drug-induced vomiting. A large number of drugs can induce central vomiting, but the most important are morphine and other narcotic drugs, and volatile anaesthetic agents. As these act on the CTZ it is logical to treat vomiting due to these agents with a phenothiazine; promethazine, prochlorperazine or triethylperazine are satisfactory choices. Post-anaesthetic vomiting is caused by the emetic effects of the volatile agent and the premedication, if this includes an opiate. The addition of atropine or hyoscine to the premedication counters the effects of both of these agents, but the duration of action of the anticholinergic may not be long enough to extend into the post-anaesthetic period. In this case an injection of a phenothiazine is the most appropriate treatment.

Metabolic vomiting. The vomiting accompanying diabetic ketoacidosis, uraemia, deep X-ray therapy or antimitotic drugs can be counteracted by phenothiazines, although anticholinergics are often equally effective. Metoclopramide is also effective (see below).

Vomiting of pregnancy. Nausea and vomiting during the first trimester is very common and is probably related to the rapid rise in circulating oestrogens. Phenothiazines may be used if vomiting becomes frequent. Thiethylperazine suppositories may be of value. Cyclizine and meclozine should be avoided because of their possible teratogenic effects. Dicyclomine is frequently used, although it has not been proven to be totally free from teratogenic potential. Pyridoxine is included in some propriety preparations on the grounds that pyridoxine deficiency can cause vomiting, but there is no evidence that it is of any value.

Motion sickness. Excessive vestibular stimulation can lead to vomiting, especially in children. In predisposed subjects antiemetic drugs should be used prophylactically, taken 1 hour before starting the journey. Anticholinergics and antihistamines are the most effective drugs, phenothiazines being of less value. Hyoscine, cyclizine and meclozine are the most popular, the first being the most powerful. Promethazine is also effective, but is more sedative. Dry mouth, blurred vision and sedation are the usual price to pay for suppression of travel sickness.

Ménière's disease. The vertigo and vomiting of this condition result from excessive stimulation of vestibular pathways by disease of the labyrinth. Anti-emetic drugs can be given prophylactically to reduce the severity of the attacks, but their effectiveness is difficult to assess. The choice of drug should be as for motion sickness. In prolonged attacks the sedative effects of prochlorperazine or promethazine may be of value, quite apart from any anti-emetic properties which they possess. These drugs are often used prophylactically, although as anti-emetics they are not as effective as anticholinergics or antihistamines. Brain stem vascular disease can produce symptoms similar to those of Ménière's disease, and they should be treated in the same manner.

Peripheral vomiting. Stimulation of autonomic afferent fibres from the thoracic and abdominal viscera can induce vomiting, e.g. following a myocardial infarction, from ingestion of a gastric irritant, or from peptic ulceration. Centrally-acting anti-emetics are of little value in these conditions. Sometimes, however, vomiting is caused partly by an opiate and partly by the condition for which it is being given, e.g. myocardial infarction, and in this case a phenothiazine anti-emetic will be of value.

Antispasmodics may be useful in some cases of peripheral vomiting. Dicyclomine, for instance, is effective in infantile vomiting and colic. Metoclopramide seems to have both central and peripheral actions. It acts on the CTZ, and it has therefore been recommended for treatment of metabolic, post-irradiation and post-anaesthetic vomiting. It also stimulates gastric smooth muscle, possibly by sensitizing the muscle to acetylcholine, thereby promoting gastric emptying and relieving pyloric spasm. Its peripheral effects are blocked by anticholinergic compounds. By dopamine receptor blockade, it can produce extra-pyramidal adverse effects, mainly of the dystonic type. Domperidone is structurally unrelated but has similar pharmacological actions.

Emetic agents

The production of vomiting is occasionally of value, especially following a drug overdose. Simple measures, such as digital stimulation of the pharynx can be effective. Ipecacuanha induces vomiting partly by a central action and partly by a local irritant one. It is slow in its action, and this limits its usefulness in drug overdosage. It is contained in small amounts in some cough linctuses, and a purified form of it, emetine, is used as an amoebicide.

Apomorphine is a semisynthetic opiate with weak analgesic and strong emetic actions. It stimulates the CTZ. Given subcutaneously it induces vomiting within a few minutes, but is too potent for clinical use.

LOCAL ANAESTHETIC AGENTS

Many drugs have local anaesthetic properties, but the only ones which are clinically useful in this respect are those which do not, at the same time, cause tissue irritation. Local anaesthesia is the result of a block of transmission in nerve fibres or their associated sensory receptors. All types of nerve are affected although small fibres are blocked first, accounting for the dissociation of pain and touch which frequently occurs during onset of, or recovery from, anaesthesia. The blockade of transmission is caused by an inhibition of the sodium influx which occurs during a propagated spike potential. This effect occurs in all excitable tissues if the local concentration is high enough. Thus local anaesthetic drugs can have antidysrhythmic and anticonvulsant properties, which are of clinical value with lignocaine. Unfortunately, toxic effects on the central nervous system also occur, producing restlessness, tremor and even convulsions.

Cocaine

This is little used now, except for surface anaesthesia of the cornea and respiratory passages (during bronchoscopy), but it is no longer the most suitable drug for these purposes. It has sympathomimetic properties by blocking reuptake of noradrenaline into nerve terminals. In the eye it causes blanching of the sclera, mydriasis and a widening of the palpebral fissure. With frequent use it can cause desquamation and ulceration of the conjunctival epithelium.

Despite its vasoconstricting properties, it is rapidly absorbed from mucous membranes and can readily produce toxic effects. It stimulates the highest centres of the brain, which accounts for its addiction potential. With chronic misuse it leads to delusions, hallucinations and paranoid ideas.

Procaine

Procaine is not suitable for surface use, for it is poorly absorbed from mucous membranes. When injected, it is rapidly hydrolysed by pseudocholinesterase in the serum, producing para-aminobenzoic acid. This substance can antagonize the bacteriostatic action of sulphonamides. It produces vasodilatation when infiltrated into tissues, and this shortens its duration of action.

Lignocaine

This is one of the most popular of local anaesthetics. It is surface-active, has little effect on blood vessel tone and is less toxic than procaine. It is metabolized in the liver, and not by pseudocholinesterase.

Bupivacaine

This is a newer drug which is now widely used, particularly for peridural analgesia in labour and in dentistry.

Others

Prilocaine is similar to lignocaine, although less toxic, and is used in dentistry. Amethocaine is powerfully surface-active and is popular in ophthalmology. Its toxicity makes it unsuitable for injection. Benzocaine is relatively weak, but finds favour in a proprietary preparation promoted for sore throats.

Clinical use

In dentistry lignocaine containing 1:80 000–200 000 adrenaline or noradrenaline is widely used. The sympathomimetic amine is added to produce vasoconstriction, making the resulting anaesthesia more reliable and of longer duration. It is preferable to avoid the use of adrenaline in patients with heart disease or hyperthyroidism, for the β-adrenergic stimulant actions of the amine can cause dysrhythmias. A noradrenaline-containing solution should be used instead, for this has much weaker β-actions. Neither catecholamine should be used in patients receiving treatment with a tricyclic antidepressant, for their pressor effects are potentiated. Felypressin, a polypeptide which produces vasoconstriction by a direct action on vascular smooth muscle, does not interact with tricyclic drugs. MAOIs do not potentiate direct acting sympathomimetic agents.

Local anaesthetics with vasoconstrictors are useful in medical work for suturing skin wounds or infiltrating the abdominal wall before incision during an operation under local anaesthesia. They should be assiduously avoided, however, for producing ring-block of an extremity, such as a finger, toe or pinna, for they can cause prolonged ischaemia which sometimes leads to gangrene of the part.

7

Psychopharmacology

At the beginning of the previous Chapter the current state of knowledge about transmitters in the CNS and their modification by drug therapy was outlined. The importance particularly of monoaminergic transmission, i.e. utilizing noradrenaline, dopamine and 5HT, was stressed. There is a growing body of opinion that a disturbance in transmission mediated by these substances is responsible for endogenous depressive illness and schizophrenia, and that drugs which are effective in treating these diseases do so by correcting the disordered transmission. These views will be further developed in this Chapter.

DRUGS IN PSYCHIATRY

Antidepressives
Considerable evidence has accumulated over recent years to support the monoamine hypothesis of the affective disorders. This hypothesis states that the level of behaviour on the depression–excitation continuum is determined by the concentration of monoamines, in certain areas of the brain which seem to be closely linked with this type of behaviour. Animal experiments in which areas of the brain are stimulated or ablated indicate that the structure most intimately concerned with emotional behaviour is the limbic system, which includes the hypothalamus, anterior thalamic nuclei, gyrus cinguli, hippocampus, amygdala and septum, and the mamillary body and fornix. These structures are rich in monoamines, and it has been reported that the concentration of 5HT is reduced in depressed patients. Experiments with drugs which modify monoaminergic transmission also support the hypothesis. Depletion of monoamine stores by reserpine leads to sedation and depression, and α-methyl p-tyrosine and α-methyldopa can have a similar effect. Reserpine depression can be antagonized by drugs which replete noradrenaline stores (e.g. levodopa) or 5HT stores (e.g. L-tryptophan) or drugs which lead to increased concentrations

of free monoamines at the nerve terminal (e.g. MAOIs and tricyclic antidepressives). MAOIs in therapeutic doses have been shown to increase the concentrations of noradrenaline and 5HT in the human brain. Although there is now abundant evidence that these substances are important for the regulation of mood and motor activity, the relative contribution which each makes is still uncertain.

Amphetamines and other stimulants
Although the amphetamines release noradrenaline and dopamine from nerve terminals the central stimulant effect of these drugs is not blocked by depletion of the granular stores by reserpine, suggesting that a direct action is more important in this respect. The stimulant action affects both mental and physical performance, but the quality of these may deteriorate even though the tasks are more speedily performed. Fatigue is delayed, while sociability and confidence increase. Other central effects are insomnia, a reduction in appetite, and hyper-reflexia, while tremor results from a direct effect on skeletal muscle. Sympathetic stimulation produces tachycardia, an increased systolic blood pressure and dryness of the mouth. When given to depressed patients amphetamines produce increased alertness and elevation of mood, but the effects are often transient and may be followed by an even deeper depression. Patients in whom depression results from an inadequate personality obtain the most benefit from amphetamines, but these are the very patients who are most likely to become dependent on them. Because of the problems of abuse they should no longer be prescribed where alternative treatment exists.

Abuse, and even therapeutic use, can be followed by a withdrawal syndrome comprising fatigue, depression, hypersomnia and an increase in rapid eye movement (REM) sleep. Prolonged use can lead to the development of a chronic psychosis, resembling paranoid schizophrenia.

Many patients receiving amphetamines experience tension and anxiety, and in order to overcome this problem barbiturates have been combined with amphetamine in several preparations (e.g. Drinamyl is a mixture of dextroamphetamine and amylobarbitone). There is evidence that these two drugs have synergistic effects which result in a greater elation and less interference with performance than is produced by either drug separately.

Other stimulant drugs include methylamphetamine, which has been given intravenously for abreaction, and methylphenidate, which has a weaker action than the amphetamines. Other related compounds, such as phenmetrazine, diethylpropion and fenfluramine are used in the treatment of obesity (Chapter 13).

MAOIs

Iproniazid, the original compound in this group, was developed as an antituberculous drug, being chemically related to isoniazid. Initial trials, in 1951, revealed a central stimulant effect. A number of compounds are now in clinical use, and can be divided into *hydrazines*, including iproniazid, isocarboxazid, phenelzine, and nialamide, and *non-hydrazines*, of which tranylcypromine is the only representative currently used in depression. This latter drug has in addition to its MAO inhibiting property a direct stimulant effect similar to that of amphetamine.

MAOIs are of most use when there is an endogenous component to the depression, but are also helpful in patients with a reactive or atypical depression, often with symptoms of an anxiety component. Psychiatric outpatients appear to respond better than do long-stay patients in mental hospitals. A delay of up to two weeks is usual between starting treatment with a hydrazine MAOI and the first signs of a response, and this appears to correlate with a gradually increasing concentration of brain monoamines during the first month of treatment. Tranylcypromine acts more quickly than the hydrazine derivatives. The dose should be gradually increased until full therapeutic dosage has been reached, and if no response is seen after four weeks the drug should be discontinued. Other antidepressive drugs should be introduced with caution during the two weeks following MAOI treatment, for interactions will occur until the enzyme has been resynthesized.

The chief disadvantage of MAOI treatment is the frequency with which adverse reactions can occur, some of which are potentially lethal.

(a) Autonomic side effects, resulting from inhibition of peripheral MAO. They include dry mouth, constipation, postural hypotension, hesitancy of micturition and delayed ejaculation.

(b) Other effects, such as water retention and oedema, and increased muscle tone and reflexes.

(c) Hepatocellular damage with hydrazine drugs, producing a mortality of up to 25 per cent of affected patients.

(d) Hypertensive crises from interaction with other drugs and foodstuffs (see p. 22). The serious nature of these crises makes it imperative that the patient is warned of these interactions, and he should be given a card to carry with him stating the drug and its dose. Many practitioners consider that the morbidity and mortality associated with the use of MAOIs is too high to justify their routine use; indeed, in some countries they are no longer marketed.

Tricyclic antidepressives (monoamine re-uptake inhibitors)
These are drugs of first choice in the treatment of depression. They are most useful in endogenous depression, in which the patient's symptoms are out of all proportion to environmental stresses. They are less effective in reactive depression, and of no value when the symptoms are the result of an inadequate personality. They are often used in conjunction with electric convulsion therapy (ECT), which in itself is still one of the most satisfactory forms of treatment for depression.

Table 7 Tricyclic and related antidepressives

Drug	Remarks
Dibenzazepine type Imipramine Desipramine ✓ Trimipramine Clomipramine Iprindole Opipramol Dibenzepin	Imipramine has a relatively small sedative effect and is therefore preferable in patients in whom there is no co-existent anxiety. Clomipramine, the chloro-derivative of imipramine, can be given intravenously and is said to be useful in obsessional and phobic disorders. Desipramine is the desmethylated derivative of imipramine.
Dibenzocycloheptene type Amitriptyline Nortriptyline Protriptyline Butriptyline Doxepin Dothiepin	Amitriptyline is sedative, therefore particularly useful in depressive illness accompanied by anxiety. Protriptyline acts in 5 to 10 days, the remainder in 10 to 14 days. Nortriptyline is the desmethylated derivative of amitriptyline.
Other Types Maprotiline Mianserin	Maprotiline resembles the tricyclic antidepressives in its pharmacological effects. Mianserin is a tetracyclic compound, and is a 5HT receptor blocking drug whose antidepressive activity was detected by its effects on the human EEG.
Viloxazine	Viloxazine is a bicyclic compound with amphetamine-like central stimulant properties.
Nomifensine	An antidepressive with an activating effect, useful in the withdrawn patient.

Chemically tricyclic compounds fall essentially into two types: (i) the imidobenzyl subgroup of the dibenzazepines (e.g. imipramine), and (ii) the dibenzocycloheptenes (e.g. amitriptyline). Although there are no marked differences in the efficacy of the many marketed tricyclic drugs, they differ in their sedative effects, adverse effects and speed of onset of action (Table 7). In patients whose depressive symptoms are accompanied by anxiety, a sedative compound such as amitriptyline, nortriptyline or doxepin should be used. If taken in a single dose last thing at night they will help the patient with insomnia. Tricyclic antidepressive drugs are most likely to help those in whom physical symptoms, psychomotor slowing and disturbed thought content are prominent.

In general, there is a 10– 14 day delay between starting treatment and the appearance of an antidepressive response. Although this may be partly explained on pharmacokinetic grounds, there are other factors involved which are not fully understood. Following a single dose of a tricyclic drug to normal volunteers, it is possible to demonstrate a blockade of the pressor response to tyramine (due to uptake blockade) within an hour or two of administration and therefore it is likely that pharmacological effects other than this may be involved in their antidepressive effect. Some compounds, e.g. imipramine, selectively block noradrenaline uptake, whereas others, e.g. clomipramine, are more active on the re-uptake of 5HT, but this difference does not appear to influence their clinical use. L-Tryptophan has been used in conjunction with tricyclics to enhance the build-up of 5HT, but its value is controversial.

Both imipramine and amitriptyline are desmethylated to active metabolites, desipramine and nortriptyline respectively, and these may accumulate to attain plasma concentrations greater than those of the parent drugs. These compounds are extensively bound both to tissue and plasma proteins, and therefore have a large apparent volume of distribution, and are eliminated slowly from the body. It takes up to 10 days for steady state to be reached after starting treatment, and it will take a similar time for the compounds to be eliminated. Monoamine oxidase inhibitors should not, therefore, be given to a patient for two weeks after withdrawal of a tricyclic drug if the danger of an interaction is to be avoided.

Once steady state has been reached, the plasma concentration of these drugs appears to be a useful guide to therapy. Carefully controlled studies have shown that an optimum antidepressive effect is seen at intermediate plasma levels, lower or higher concentrations being associated with a poorer response. At low levels, the concentration of the drug in the brain may be inadequate while at high levels it possible that the therapeutic effect is blocked by some other pharmacological action, e.g. anticholinergic effects. If this relationship between serum level and effect is confirmed, it will become important to monitor plasma levels because failure due to overdosing may be difficult to distinguish from that due to underdosing. Furthermore, tricyclic drugs show a wide pharmacokinetic variation between subjects. If monitoring becomes routine, it would be of advantage to prescribe desipramine or nortriptyline rather than their parent drugs because only one active substance will then need to be measured. These two compounds are entirely satisfactory for routine use. The relationship between plasma level and effect has been most thoroughly investigated for nortriptyline, the optimum therapeutic response appearing at levels of 200 to 600 nmol/1 (50 to 160 ng/ml).

The tricyclic antidepressives are useful also for the treatment of nocturnal enuresis, but are less helpful when the enuresis occurs during the day. Full antidepressive doses must be used.

Adverse effects with these drugs are frequent:

(a) Autonomic side-effects result partly from the blockade of noradrenaline uptake in sympathetic nerve terminals and partly from anticholinergic properties which these compounds possess. Tachycardia, palpitations, postural hypotension, dry mouth, hesitancy of micturition, and ocular effects, such as impaired accommodation, mydriasis and aggravation of narrow-angle glaucoma, are common.

(b) Electrocardiographic changes (flattened T waves, prolongation of the $Q-T$ interval and $S-T$ depression) and dysrhythmias have been noted both with imipramine and with amitriptyline. The latter drug has been shown to produce an increase in the incidence of sudden death in patients with pre-existing cardiac disease.

(c) Jaundice of the cholestatic type occurs rarely, particularly with iprindole.

(d) Central nervous effects include an increase in physiological tremor, drowsiness, disorientation, psychosis and hallucinations. Tricyclic drugs have a convulsant action and should be prescribed with caution in epilepsy.

(e) Dangerous interaction can occur between these drugs and the MAOIs. However, cautious combined use of the two types of compound has been advocated by some for the treatment of resistant depression.

(f) Tricyclic antidepressives potentiate the actions of directly-acting sympathomimetic amines. Dangerous hypertension can occur if local anaesthetic solutions containing a sympathomimetic vasoconstrictor substance are used in patients on tricyclics (pp. 28, 90).

Depression plus hypertension

An association between these two conditions is important in two respects:

(i) Some antihypertensive drugs can cause depression by interfering with monoamine metabolism in the brain. This is especially true of the Rauwolfia alkaloids, but is not uncommon with α-methyldopa and clonidine. A hypertensive patient with a history of depression should not be treated with either of these drugs. The other antihypertensive drugs only rarely cause depressive symptoms.

(ii) Sometimes both conditions coexist in a patient, and each is serious enough to require treatment. Unfortunately, the tricyclic antidepressives antagonize many antihypertensive drugs (e.g. guanethidine, bethanidine, debrisoquine, clonidine, but not α-methyldopa) by blocking their uptake into sympathetic nerve terminals, and MAOIs can reverse the action of reserpine and α-methyldopa causing release of catecholamines peripherally and centrally, leading to hypertension and hallucinations. In these patients, the hypertension can be treated with propranolol, a thiazide diuretic or a drug like prazosin, none of which interacts significantly with antidepressive drugs.

Antipsychotic drugs
Whereas barbiturates have a generalized depressant effect on the central nervous system, phenothiazines and other tranquillizers exert a more selective action on certain structures which are concerned in the regulation of behaviour and wakefulness. The reticular activating system includes those parts of the midbrain reticular formation and thalamic nuclei which give rise to diffuse cortical projections concerned in maintaining a state of alertness in the cerebral cortex. Phenothiazines are selectively concentrated in these structures and block EEG arousal produced in experimental animals by sensory stimulation, possibly by an effect on the sensory collateral fibres entering the recticular formation from the lemniscal pathways. Monoamines are present in these colaterals and it may be relevant that phenothiazines block noradrenergic, dopaminergic and tryptaminergic receptors in the CNS.

Phenothiazines depress the activity of the hypothalamus and other limbic structures, most of which are particularly rich in monoamines. Their tranquillizing and antipsychotic effects, as well as their adverse effects on the extrapyramidal system correlate best with their dopamine receptor blocking properties, and therefore much attention has been devoted to the distribution of dopamine in the brain. Two pathways are particularly rich in the transmitter, the nigro-striate pathway ascending from the brain-stem to the corpus striatum (p. 66), and the mesolimbic system ascending to the nucleus accumbens and other frontal limbic structures. It seems likely that the antipsychotic effects are due to dopamine receptor blockade in the latter system whereas the extra-pyramidal effects are caused by blockade of the nigro-striate pathway. These discoveries, together with the observation that amphetamines (which stimulate central dopamine receptors) can produce a dose-related schizophreniform psychosis, have led to the hypothesis that schizophrenia may be due either to a hypersensitivity of mesolimbic dopamine receptors or to the lack of a transmitter which is normally antagonistic to dopamine. Blocking dopamine receptors would restore the correct balance and alleviate the symptoms, although a similar effect in the striatum would independently produce extrapyramidal effects.

On the other hand, there is evidence that GABA and its synthetic enzyme, glutamic acid decarboxylase, may be deficient in the nucleus accumbens and thalamus of schizophrenic patients and it has been suggested that this deficiency may be a biochemical characteristic underlying the disorder. It is of interest in this regard that butyrophenone drugs inhibit GABA uptake into presynaptic terminals, and their potency in this correlates well with their effectiveness as antipsychotic drugs.

Phenothiazines

The first useful phenothiazine to be introduced was promethazine, which is now used only as an antihistamine and sedative drug. This was followed by chlorpromazine and subsequently a large number of related compounds. (Table 8). They can be classified into three groups according the nature of a side chain on the phenothiazine nucleus:

(i) aliphatic side chain (dimethylaminopropyl) derivatives,
(ii) piperazine derivatives, and
(iii) piperidine derivatives.

All these compounds have, to varying extents, blocking actions at α-adrenergic, dopaminergic, tryptaminergic and cholinergic receptors, as well as having antihistamine properties. Those derivatives with a dimethylaminopropyl or piperazine side chain have marked α-adrenolytic and weak anticholinergic actions, whereas those with a piperidine side chain have the reverse. The latter derivatives produce less extrapyramidal disturbance than those of the other two groups, possibly because their greater anticholinergic effect counteracts the effect of dopamine blockade, in the same manner as atropine-like drugs have been used for treating Parkinson's disease (p. 66).

Table 8 Antipsychotic drugs

Drug	Remarks
Phenothiazines	
Chlorpromazine	Dimethylaminopropyl derivatives. Chlorpromazine is
Promazine	standard drug, but is very sedative.
Prochlorperazine	Piperazine derivatives. Prochlorperazine is equivalent
Trifluoperazine	to chlorpromazine, but is less sedative. Useful also as
Perphenazine	an enti-emetic. Fluphenazine enanthate and decanoate
Fluphenazine	are long-acting depot preparations for antipsychotic
Pericyazine	maintenance therapy. Thiopropazate is used in dys-
Thiopropazate	kinesias. Pericyazine has been recommended for use
Methotrimeprazine	in character disorders.
Thioridazine	Piperidine derivative. Few extrapyramidal adverse effects.
Thioxanthenes	
Chlorprothixene	Analogues of chlorpromazine, thioproperazine and
Thiothixene	fluphenazine respectively. Flupenthixol decanoate is
Flupenthixol	depot preparation.
Butyrophenones	
Haloperidol	As effective as phenothiazines but extrapyramidal
Trifluperidol	adverse effects frequent.
Benperidol	
Indoles	
Oxypertine	Equal to phenothiazines as antipsychotic.
Diphenylbutylpiperidines	
Pimozide	For maintenance therapy, pimozide once daily
Fluspirilene	(orally), fluspirilene once weekly (intramuscularly).

The development of the phenothiazines represented the first major advance in the drug treatment of psychiatric disease, and their introduction in 1955 has dramatically reversed the steady increase in the number of patients requiring admission to a long-stay mental hospital. Their calming and antipsychotic properties make them particularly useful in treating schizophrenia. They can improve the blunted affect, withdrawal, thought disorder and secondary symptoms such as hallucinations and delusions, and reduce hyperactivity and aggression. It has been suggested that they 'normalize' thinking. Piperazine derivatives are the most potent weight for weight, and because they have a less sedative effect they are preferable in the withdrawn patient. Chlorpromazine has the greatest sedative effect and is the drug of choice in treating violent patients. In lower dosage phenothiazines can be useful in anxiety states and psychosomatic disorders. Long-acting preparations, e.g. fluphenazine enanthate or decanoate, are valuable in reducing the relapse rate in schizophrenic patients, but their use is associated with a high incidence of adverse effects, particularly depression and extrapyramidal disturbances.

Other conditions for which phenothiazines are used inlcude:

1. Nausea and vomiting: chlorpromazine, prochlorperazine and trifluoperazine are the most used in this respect. Another phenothiazine, thiethylperazine, is used exclusively for this purpose (p. 87).

2. Travel sickness: promethazine, which possesses little anti-psychotic activity, is useful in motion sickness, probably related to its anticholinergic actions.

3. Allergic reactions, e.g. acute urticaria and hay fever: the powerful antihistaminic effects of promethazine are most used for this purpose.

4. Pruritus: this is sometimes caused by histamine release in the skin, e.g. in acute urticaria, but in pruritus associated with jaundice it is unrelated to histamine release. Phenothiazines are anti-pruritic probably by a central sedative action in addition to antihistaminic effects. Promethazine and trimeprazine are widely used.

5. Pain: severe pain, particularly in terminal disease, can often be controlled much better by addition of a phenothiazine.

6. Insomnia: the sedative and hypnotic effects of these compounds, particularly promethazine, can be useful.

7. Hiccough.

8. Dyskinesias: although phenothiazines can cause dyskinesias (see below, thiopropazate may be useful in controlling them (p. 71).

Adverse effects are many because phenothiazines have numerous different pharmacological actions:

(a) Peripheral autonomic effects resulting from blockade of α-adrenergic and cholinergic receptors. Postural hypotension from peripheral vasodilation is troublesome, particularly when the drug is administered parenterally. On the other hand, phenothiazines can reverse the hypotensive action of sympathetic neurone blocking drugs by preventing their uptake into the nerve terminals. Anticholinergic actions produce dry mouth, disturbance of accommodation, constipation and hesitancy of micturition. Quinidine-like effects on the heart are occasionally seen, producing prolongation of the $Q-T$ interval and T wave changes.

(b) Central effects resulting from modification of monoaminergic transmission. Extrapyramidal syndromes are frequently produced when high doses of phenothiazines are used for treating schizophrenia. Indeed, it is thought by some that treatment is inadequate until mild extrapyramidal disturbances are evident. Aliphatic side chain derivatives frequently produce Parkinsonism while piperazine derivatives more often cause dyskinesias. Piperidine derivatives, as mentioned above, rarely produce extra-pyramidal effects although tardive (i.e. late onset) dyskinesias can occur. Phenothiazine-induced dyskinesias occur more often in the young, whereas Parkinsonism is the usual syndrome produced in the elderly. Because of the frequency of these side-effects, it is the practice in some centres to prescribe simultaneously an antiParkinsonian drug when phenothiazines are required in high doses. This is not good practice, however; extrapyramidal effects are better treated when they occur. This will avoid the risk of central and peripheral anticholinergic adverse effects and will prevent a drug interaction in which the antiParkinsonian drug can induce the metabolism of the phenothiazine. Endocrine disturbances, such as hyperprolactinaemia, galactorrhoea, and amenorrhoea, accompanied by a reduced urinary excretion of sex hormones and their metabolites, result probably from dopamine receptor blockade in the hypothalamus. Hypothermia is also due to a disturbance of hypothalamic function. Phenothiazines also have a convulsant action, the mechanism of which is unknown, and therefore they should be prescribed with caution in epilepsy.

(c) A variety of other effects, including skin rashes, pigmentation, photosensitivity, agranulocytosis, retinopathy and granular deposits in the lens and cornea. Cholestatic jaundice is a dose-independent hypersensitivity reaction, particularly to chlorpromazine, and occasionally leads to permanent liver damage.

Butyrophenones

Haloperidol, trifluperidol and benperidol have proved useful in the management of psychotic patients, in particular those with a manic psychosis although recent trials have shown that they have no advantage over chlorpromazine. Weight for weight they are more potent than chlorpromazine. Another member of this group, droperidol has been used in combination with an analgesic, phenoperidine, for producing 'neuroleptanalgesia', a twilight state in which the patient can undergo a surgical procedure without pain, and subsequently have total amnesia for the event.

Because they are only weak antihistaminics, and almost completely lack anticholinergic and α-adrenolytic effects in therapeutic doses, they infrequently produce autonomic adverse effects. Blockade of dopamine receptors frequently leads to dose-related extrapyramidal side-effects, as with phenothiazines. Depressive reactions, loss of appetite, and a syndrome including sweating, dehydration and hyperthermia can occur. Leukopenia and liver damage are occasionally seen.

Other antipsychotic drugs

The thioxanthene compounds (Table 8) are chemically closely related to the phenothiazines and appear to have similar pharmacological effects to their analogues. For maintenance therapy, flupenthixol decanoate is less likely to cause depression than its fluphenazine equivalent. Oxypertine also appears equal in efficacy to phenothiazines in schizophrenia, but in lower doses it is useful in treating anxiety states. Pimozide and fluspirilene offer the advantage of once daily and once weekly administration respectively.

Anti-anxiety drugs

The anti-anxiety drugs differ from the phenothiazines and butyrophenones in that they have no antipsychotic activity, do not importantly affect monoamine receptors peripherally or centrally, thus producing no autonomic or extrapyramidal effects, and are more active at a spinal level, reducing transmission in polysynaptic pathways and lessening spasticity.

Benzodiazepines

The most widely used minor tranquillizers are the benzodiazepines. Chlordiazepoxide was first marketed in the mid-1960's and rapidly became popular despite its relatively mild tranquillizing effect. It was followed by diazepam, nitrazepam, medazepam, oxazepam, lorazepam, flurazepam, temazepam and potassium clorazepate. All of these compounds are 1,4-benzodiazepines and are closely interrelated metabolically. As can be seen from Figure 12, the major metabolite of diazepam is N-desmethyldiazepam (nordiazepam), which is pharmacologically active. The metabolites of these two compounds are temazepam and oxazepam respectively, which are marketed compounds lacking active metabolites. Potassium clorazepate is a pro-drug for N-desmethyldiazepam, and medazepam is rapidly converted to diazepam.

Because of the close interrelationships between these drugs, it can be questioned whether they differ much one from another. In terms of their effects on receptor sites, they probably do not. Current research suggests that they have a high affinity for specific 'benzodiazepine receptors' which facilitate the effects of the inhibitory transmitter GABA in the nervous system; these receptors are found in high concentration in the cerebral cortex, midbrain and limbic structures. So potent are some of the newer ben-

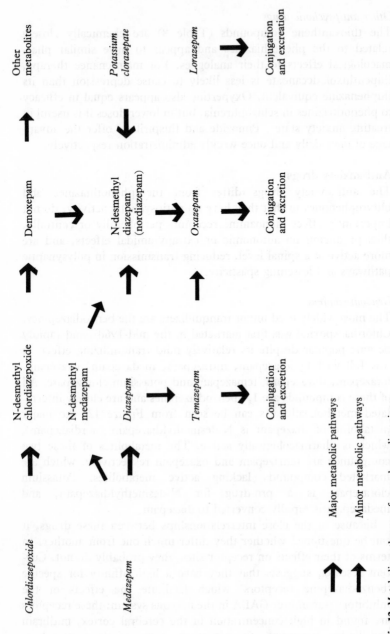

Fig 12 Metabolic pathways of some benzodiazepines

Table 9 Elimination half-lives of some common benzodiazepine drugs

Parent drug	Half-life(h)	Major active metabolite(s)	Half-life(h)
Diazepam	20–45	N-desmethyldiazepam	50–100
Clorazepate	Very short	N-desmethyldiazepam	50–100
Medazepam	Short	Diazepam	20–45
		N-desmethyldiazepam	
Chlordiazepoxide	10–20	N-desmethylchlordiazepoxide	10–20
		Demoxepam	20–70
		N-desmethyldiazepam	50–100
Oxazepam	10–20	–	
Temazepam	5–12	–	
Lorazepam	10–20	–	
Nitrazepam	20–40	–	
Flurazepam	Short	N-desalkylflurazepam	50–100
Triazolam	2–4	7-α-hydroxyderivative	3–6
Clobazam	10–30	N-desmethylclobazam	30–50
Clonazepam	20–40	–	

zodiazepine compounds that the presence of an endogenous ligand (with a specificity for benzodiazepine receptors resembling that of endorphins for opiate receptors) has been sought. A likely candidate with extraordinary potency has been identified, ethyl- β-carboline-3-carboxylate.

In vivo, however, the effects of the various 1,4-benzodiazepines differ in time course because their pharmacokinetic properties differ. Those that have the common major metabolite N-desmethyldiazepam, namely diazepam, medazepam and clorazepate are indistinguishable because the metabolite is pharmacologically active and has a half-life which exceeds those of the parent compounds (Table 9). When diazepam is given chronically, serum levels of N-desmethyldiazepam are on average twice as high as those of diazepam itself, and therefore the pharmacokinetics of the metabolite are more important in determining the time course of the drug's effect. These are therefore long-acting preparations and are suitable as anti-anxiety drugs but not as hypnotics.

Oxazepam, temazepam and lorazepam do not have active metabolites but are conjugated and excreted. Their half-lives are shorter and they can therefore be used when a less prolonged effect is required. Temazepam is marketed as a short-acting hypnotic, for which purpose it is very suitable. Oxazepam penetrates the blood-brain barrier more slowly and is less suitable for this purpose.

Triazolam is a benzodiazepine derivative with a triazole structure. It is potent and has a half-life of only 2–4 hours. Although it has an active metabolite (Table 9) this also has a short half-life and therefore triazolam might be valuable as a short-acting hypnotic drug.

Clobazam is a 1,5 benzodiazepine which is claimed to possess an antianxiety effect without psychomotor impairment, but further assessment is needed before its place is certain.

Benzodiazepine drugs have five main uses:

1. As antianxiety compounds. There is evidence that they act selectively on the limbic system, in particular the septum, amygdala and hippocampus, and many clinical trials have demonstrated their superiority over barbiturates. In general, a longer acting drug would appear to be most suitable for this purpose, although those with a shorter half-life, e.g. oxazepam and lorazepam, have also been promoted as antianxiety preparations.

Benzodiazepines have become one of the most widely used groups of drugs in the world, and some have suggested too widely used. Although tranquillizer therapy may be fully justified when the response to life's stresses and strains is pathological, it is arguable whether normal feelings of anxiety, which may improve rather than impair performance, need treatment. Furthermore, such therapy is not without its risks. There is accumulating evidence that both psychological and physical dependence to benzodiazepine drugs can occur. The latter is presumably due to a gradual change in the sensitivity of the benzodiazepine receptor site, leading to tolerance to the pharmacological effects of these compounds. It has been clearly shown that chronic use is associated with a gradual diminution in their hypnotic and antiepileptic effects, and the same is presumably true of their antianxiety action. Certainly, a clear-cut withdrawal syndrome can occur on abruptly stopping chronic benzodiazepine therapy, and includes insomnia, anxiety, tremulousness, muscle tension and twitchings, distorted perception (particularly hypersensitivity to light and sound), illusiory phenomena, and seizures. The appearance of these symptoms on stopping or reducing long-term therapy has led many patients to continue unnecessary treatment. The withdrawal syndrome is particularly severe when high doses have been given, e.g. 30 mg. or more of diazepam daily; sometimes the tolerance which occurs with repeated administration leads to an escalation of dosage far exceeding the recommendations in the data sheet. Therefore, if a benzodiazepine drug is prescribed for anxiety it should be given in as low a dosage and for as short a time as possible. Furthermore, the patient should be warned against increasing the dose on his own initiative, or stopping the drug suddenly.

One advantage which benzodiazepines possess over other CNS

depressant drugs is their safety in overdosage. Suicide attempts seldom succeed, even with massive doses, unless combined with another substance such as alcohol. Sedation, tiredness, muscle weakness, ataxia and diplopia are common adverse effects and, as with other tranquillizers and sedatives, driving performance is impaired and patients should be warned of this. Confusion can occur in the elderly, and this may be due to a reduced rate of metabolism, but also to an increased sensitivity of the ageing brain to depressant substances.

2. *As soporific drugs* given intravenously preoperatively or during dental and endoscopic procedures.

3. *As hypnotic drugs* (see p. 110).

4. *As antispasticity drugs* (p. 81) or to relieve muscle spasm associated with anxiety.

5. *As anticonvulsant drugs* given intravenously in status epilepticus (p. 77), or chronically in the management of myoclonic epilepsies (p. 76).

Other minor tranquillizers
Meprobamate has been widely used in the treatment of anxiety, particularly in the United States, where the trade name Miltown became a household word. Since the introduction of the benzodiazepines, however, its popularity has declined. Drowsiness and hypersensitivity reactions occur frequently, as do tolerance and dependence.

Several other anti-anxiety drugs are available, such as prothipendyl, benzoctamine and hydroxyzine, but they are less effective than the benzodiazepines.

Lithium
Although lithium salts were used in clinical medicine many years ago, they fell into disrepute because of their toxic side-effects. Recently they have been reintroduced and have proved useful in the management of manic-depressive psychosis, and possibly in some patients with unipolar endogenous depression. Lithium calms manic patients and also maintains a normal mood as long as the drug is continued. Careful regulation of the dose is necessary, and frequent measurement of the plasma lithium concentration should be performed. This should be kept between 0·8 and 1·2 mmol/litre.

The drug is usually given as the carbonate or citrate. Lithium ions behave as sodium ions in excitable tissues, but cause a depression of the resting potential and spike potential. They also enhance the uptake of noradrenaline into nerve terminals and alter its metabolism in such a way as to make less of the transmitter available at the receptor. The effects on brain catecholamines are more likely to be relevant to their therapeutic effect than changes in polarization of the nerve cell.

Adverse effects are common. Tremor is almost invariable, and can be used as a clinical guide to dosage. Serum levels above 1·2 to 1·4 mmol/litre produce diarrhoea and vomiting. Tinnitus, drowsiness, ataxia, blurred vision, thirst and polyuria occur at higher levels, with confusion, nystagmus and fits when the level reaches 3 mmol/litre. Above 4 mmol/litre the outcome is usually fatal. The most serious toxic effect is on the kidney, producing a water-losing nephritis. When intoxication occurs withdrawal of lithium therapy is essential. Addition of sodium chloride to the diet has been recommended to hasten elimination of lithium, but in practice the effect is small. Goitre, sometimes accompanied by severe hypothyroidism, has been observed during lithium treatment more frequently than would be expected by chance.

Psychotomimetic drugs

These include synthetic lysergic acid derivatives, of which the diethylamide (LSD) is the most important, mescaline, which comes from the Mexican peyote cactus, and psilocybin, which is extracted from several species of mushroom. The psychic syndromes produced by these three compounds closely resemble each other. In normal man they induce:

1. Autonomic effects which are almost invariable and result from central stimulation of autonomic pathways. They include blurred vision, a rise in blood pressure, palpitations, and frequency of micturition. Other somatic symptoms occur, such as nausea, vomiting, tremulousness and ataxia.

2. Changes in mood. Anxiety and fear are common. Dramatic swings in mood can occur, from profound depression one moment to hilarious laughter the next. Euphoria, hypomania and paranoia sometimes occur.

3. Changes in thought processes, such as difficulty in concentration, indecision, introspection and slipshod thinking.

4. Perceptual changes are not a constant feature, but are frequently seen. Vivid visual distortions or even hallucinations can occur. Auditory and tactile changes are less frequent. Distortion of body image and time sense are occasionally produced.

The pharmacological basis of these effects is uncertain. LSD is a powerful 5HT antagonist, but psilocybin is only weak in this respect, and mescalin has no anti-5HT effects at all. Furthermore, other lysergic acid derivatives are potent 5HT antagonists but have no psychotomimetic activity. It has been suggested that these drugs stimulate afferent collaterals feeding into the ascending reticular formation, which might account for changes in perception.

They have no generally accepted therapeutic uses, although they have been tried in a variety of mental diseases, and have been used for abreaction and as an adjunct to psychoanalysis. The dangers of treatment with psychotomimetic drugs, even in single doses, are substantial. Prolonged states of depression or anxiety may occur, sometimes so severe that the subject may become suicidal. Psychotic behaviour developing during the stage of acute intoxication may make the subject a danger to himself or others. Prolonged psychotic illness may ensue. The foolhardiness of experimenting with these drugs is obvious.

HYPNOTICS AND SEDATIVES

It is customary to subdivide central depressant drugs into hypnotics, sedatives and tranquillizers, partly on clinical usage of the various drugs and partly on their neuropharmacological effects in animals. Drugs which have a general depressant effect on the CNS, such as the barbiturates, have been much used as hypnotics. Drugs which seem to be more selective in their effects on central structures, acting particularly on the ascending reticular formation and limbic system, have been promoted as tranquillizers which are claimed to reduce anxiety without producing sedation. In clinical practice, however, the relevance of this classification is less obvious (see below).

Before prescribing a hypnotic the reason for the insomnia should first be sought. If pain is the cause an analgesic should be prescribed, either alone, or in combination with a hypnotic. The latter given alone often has an 'antianalgesic' effect, making the patient with pain even more restless. The only exception to this is when the pain is accompanied by considerable anxiety. Here a sedative or tranquillizer may be helpful. In patients with respiratory failure further desensitization of the respiratory centre to an already elevated P CO_2 can precipitate CO_2 narcosis. Respiratory failure can occur in a patient in status asthmaticus, who may be critically dependent upon a raised PCO_2 to maintain respiratory drive.

Hypnotics, like tranquillizers, are amongst the most abused of drugs, both by the practitioner and by the patient. Barbiturates alone account for over half of all deaths from drug overdosage, and this reflects largely the ease with which a prescription for these compounds can be obtained. Tolerance, addiction and characteristic withdrawal symptoms have been reported with every known hypnotic, although barbiturates are probably the most potent in this respect. Withdrawal symptoms include convulsions, delerium, restlessness and insomnia accompanied by a rebound increase in REM sleep. The latter symptoms can persist for several weeks after an overdose or on withdrawal of a regular intake of the drug, and can reinforce the patient's opinion that he cannot sleep without a nightly dose of hypnotic. Inadvertently, a sympathetic practitioner prescribing a hypnotic to tide a patient over a crisis may start a lifelong habit which is not easily broken. Hypnotics should never be prescribed without serious thought about the long-term consequences, and can usually be avoided by sensible discussion. Should one be considered necessary, a benzodiazepine compound should be chosen. Barbiturates should now be considered obsolete for all but intravenous anaesthesia and epilepsy.

Benzodiazepines

Although, ideally, a hypnotic effect is an undesirable property of a tranquillizer, all the benzodiazepines have marked hypnotic actions in higher doses. Pharmacological tranquillization and hypnosis are certainly not as distinct as some promotional literature would have us believe, and any of the marketed benzodiazepine compounds can be used for night time sedation.

However, in order to achieve rapid induction of sleep and a minimum of hangover effect the next day, a benzodiazepine which is quickly absorbed and which has a short elimination half-life should be selected. The drug which has been most widely used as an hypnotic is nitrazepam, but this fails to meet the ideal because it has a long half-life (Table 9). Similarly, flurazepam has a long duration of action because of the slow elimination of its major metabolite, N-desalkylflurazepam. From the pharmacokinetic point of view, temazepam or, perhaps triazolam, would be selected, but both these drugs are expensive. The choice, however, is determined partly by the frequency with which the hypnotic will be used. For occasional use, a drug with a long half-life may not be unacceptable, but with nightly use these compounds (or their active metabolites) may accumulate and produce continuing day-time sedation. Tolerance, however, is a factor which needs to be taken into account. With repeated administration, the hypnotic effect (and the hangover effect) diminishes until eventually only a trivial pharmacological action remains. Rebound insomnia may, of course, occur when attempts are made to stop the drug.

One major advantage of benzodiazepines over the barbiturates is safety in overdosage. However, respiratory depression can occur, and they should therefore be avoided in patients with chronic respiratory disease. Unlike barbiturates, benzodiazepines do not induce liver enzymes, and are therefore safe in combination with oral anticoagulants.

Barbiturates

These compounds have traditionally been divided into long-, medium-, short- and ultrashort-acting drugs. The latter, by virtue of their high lipid solubility, are used as induction agents in general anaesthesia but their effect is brief because they are redistributed to other tissues, mainly fat and muscle, and they are subsequently gradually metabolized by the liver. The short- and medium-acting drugs are also degraded by the liver, and although their rates of absorption and metabolism vary slightly, this is of little practical significance. Amylobarbitone, butobarbitone, cyclobarbitone, pentobarbitone and quinalbarbitone are all similar in action as hypnotics, but their use has been largely superceded by the benzodiazepine drugs.

Barbiturates are strictly contraindicated in acute intermittent porphyria. Liver disease can impair barbiturate metabolism, although in practice the effect is not great. The powerful liver enzyme inducing property of these compounds can lead to many drug interactions, of which the most dangerous is that with oral anticoagulants. Long-term use of barbiturates leads to the development of considerable tolerance, partly resulting from accelerated metabolism by liver enzyme induction, but partly from a chemical tolerance at a cellular level.

Elderly patients may be intolerant of barbiturates, becoming confused and restless, but younger patients can sometimes also be affected in this way, leading to amnesia and repetition of the dose. Although a number of overdoses are claimed to have occurred in this way it is probably seldom true. However, patients should not keep their tablets at the bedside.

Chloral hydrate

Although this compound was introduced just over 100 years ago it is still a useful hypnotic, especially in the young and the old. It is available only in liquid form, as the crystalline substance is hygroscopic. It is bitter to taste and irritant to the stomach. Combination of chloral hydrate with alcohol produces a potent central depressant, and this is the basis of a 'Mickey Finn'. It is largely converted by the liver to trichloroethanol, which is itself a potent hypnotic. It is one of the safest, cheapest and least toxic of hypnotics, although addiction has occasionally been reported.

Tablet forms of chloral have been introduced by esterification (Triclofos) and by combining it with phenazone (dichloralphenazone). The latter combination is reversed by liver enzymes, and the phenazone which is released can occasionally cause rashes and agranulocytosis. Phenazone, also called antipyrine, has been used as an analgesic, but is now obsolete.

Chloral preparations interact with oral anticoagulants, but in a different way from barbiturates. One of the metabolites, trichloroacetic acid, displaces the anticoagulant from its binding with plasma proteins, increasing its effect as well as its rate of elimination.

Other drugs

Paraldehyde has been much used as a hypnotic, or as a sedative in disturbed patients, but its physical properties have caused it to lose favour. It is well absorbed when taken by mouth, but it is unpalatable. It is usually injected intramuscularly, but is irritant, can damage the sciatic nerve when injected badly, and causes sterile abscesses. It is exhaled in the breath, producing a penetrating and objectionable odour. Despite these disadvantages it is relatively safe. It has useful anticonvulsant activity in status epilepticus (p. 78).

Glutethimide is a close relative of the barbiturates, and may be even more likely to cause a fatal outcome in overdosage. Aminoglutethimide, introduced as a hypnotic was found to cause a block in adrenal steroid synthesis, but this has been put to use therapeutically in Cushing's syndrome.

Methylpentynol is a short-acting drug, taken as a liquid in capsules. Unpleasant belching may occur the following day. It has been a popular sedative in dentistry.

Methaqualone resembles the barbiturates in its action, but has few side-effects. In combination with diphenhydramine (Mandrax) rapid hypnosis is produced, but this proprietary preparation has become popular with addicts. Overdosage is often accompanied by convulsions, which are due to the diphenhydramine.

Promethazine, the phenothiazine antihistamine, is a long-acting hypnotic which has been found useful in children and the elderly. It is of value when early waking occurs. Trimeprazine is similar, and is popular as a preoperative sedative in children.

Alcohol is a useful, palatable and under-used hypnotic in the elderly.

Other drugs include ethchlorvynol, ethinamate, and chlormethiazole.

NARCOTIC ANALGESICS

Physiology of pain

The concept of pain as a separate modality of sensation, with its own sensory receptors, afferent fibres and ascending spinal pathways, has not been supported by recent neurophysiological research. Further theories have been based upon the electrical properties of nerve cells, and the ways in which these properties permit coding of sensory information so that common receptors and pathways may be used, but also allow decoding in higher centres. It has been recognized for some years that sensory input can be inhibited or facilitated by pathways travelling in an opposite direction to the afferent fibres, and which control transmission at the first sensory synapse. This provides a neurophysiological basis for the concept of a 'gate', which can be opened to allow information through or closed to stop it. There is some evidence that fast-conducting afferents may initiate inhibitory feedback which blocks conduction in slower afferent fibres, whereas these latter fibres can facilitate conduction. Certain pathological conditions which are characterized by pain may cause an imbalance between these two opposing forces. Non-painful sensation may become painful when the input of sensory information becomes excessive either in space or in time, or takes up a certain pattern. These changes would then cause activation of central neurones with a high threshold which are concerned with the appreciation of pain.

It is possible that centrally-acting analgesics, including opiates and some general anaesthetic agents, may act by influencing this descending (or centrifugal) control system, causing a block or change in the pattern of a potentially pain-invoking sensory input. Recent research suggests that opiate actions involve highly specific receptors in the brain, which may normally be activated by intrinsic morphine-like substances whose physiological role is that of synaptic transmission. These substances, called endorphins and enkephalins are polypeptides with amino-acid sequences corresponding with those of the C-terminal of β-lipotrophin. They are distributed widely in the CNS, but exist in particularly high concentration in the substantia gelatinosa, the zone which caps the dorsal horn of the spinal cord and is probably largely involved with the modulation of sensory information. It is likely that small cells in this zone produce enkephalins which have an important role in modifying the transfer of potentially painful sensory information to ascending pathways, i.e. acting as a 'gate' (Fig. 13).

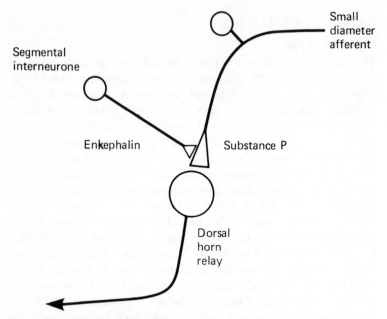

Fig. 13 Proposed scheme for inhibitory control of enkephalin-producing interneurones in the substantia gelatinosa over primary afferent fibres producing the excitatory transmitter, substance P.

β-Endorphin and methionine enkephalin can produce profound analgesia when injected intraventricularly in animals and intrathecally in man. The specific opiate antagonist, naloxone, can lower pain threshold in some people, can increase post-operative dental pain, and reverse the analgesic effect produced by a placebo and by acupuncture. These observations suggest that endorphins and enkephalins may play an important physiological role in pain control, and that narcotic analgesics act by mimicking these endogenous substances.

From the practical point of view there are two types of pain, visceral and somatic. The former is a dull, poorly localized pain, and is not helped by non-narcotic drugs, whereas the latter is sharply defined, is usually relieved by a mild analgesic and seldom requires an opiate. This, perhaps, is fortunate as there are many chronic musculoskeletal conditions which require analgesic treatment over many years. The use of opiate drugs should not be contemplated unless the painful condition is of very limited duration, e.g. postoperative, or accompanies terminal disease such as cancer, when addiction is of no concern.

Pain is a symptom of underlying pathology and is of vital diagnostic importance. Its uncritical relief is to be deplored, as a valuable sign of worsening disease will be lost. Treatment should be given only when a firm diagnosis has been made and an alternative means of assessment is available.

As in many other areas of therapeutics a placebo effect is important in the treatment of pain. One study showed that capsules containing 10 mg of morphine were only slightly superior to placebo in relieving postoperative pain, and the placebo itself gave relief in almost one third of the patients. In another study of experimental pain in fit adults, 50 mg of pethidine intramuscularly was indistinguishable from saline, and 100 mg was only slightly superior.

Pharmacology of narcotic analgesics

These compounds have effects on many different tissues, probably resulting from influencing important, but poorly understood, intracellular enzyme systems. In brief, the following pharmacological actions are seen:

(a) Central effects, including analgesia, euphoria and drowsiness. These are associated with changes in electrical activity in various parts of the brain, particularly the cerebral cortex, thalamus and reticular formation. An elevation of the pain threshold seems to occur, but, in addition, the patient's attitude and emotional response to the pain is altered. This euphoriant effect is the reason why opiates are drugs of abuse.

(b) Respiratory depresssion is produced by an effect on the respiratory centre, lowering its sensitivity to changes in PCO_2. This seems to parallel analgesic activity in the many different opiates.

(c) Depression of the cough reflex. Opiates are included in a number of cough mixtures.

(d) Nausea and vomiting particularly with morphine, resulting from stimulation of the chemoreceptor trigger zone. This occurs every time in some patients, but never in others. Larger doses of morphine inhibit vomiting by an action on the emetic centre.

(e) Miosis, from stimulation of the parasympathetic outflow responsible for pupillo-constriction. Pethidine and its analogues lack this effect.

(f) Increase in smooth muscle tone and a reduction in its motility, causing constipation, spasm of the sphincter of Oddi and bronchoconstriction.

(g) Hypotension, from depression of ganglionic transmission, producing vasodilatation.

(h) Histamine release occurs occasionally, especially with morphine, causing urticaria and pruritus.

Individual compounds. A wide variety of compounds are available, some being naturally-occurring alkaloids and others semisynthetic or synthetic. Discussion will be confined to the more important representatives. Essentially they can be divided into four groups:

(a) Morphine group, including morphine itself, the semisynthetic opiate diamorphine (heroin), and the synthetic opioid compounds, levorphanol, dextromoramide, phenazocine and pentazocine, which closely resemble morphine in structure and actions. Morphine is still the most used of these drugs but it frequently produces nausea and vomiting. Diamorphine is preferred by some on the grounds that it less often causes these effects, and also rarely constipates. It has less tendency to produce hypotension and for this reason is often chosen in patients who have had a myocardial infarction, for the mortality in this condition is directly related to the occurrence of hypotension. It also produces more euphoria, and this may be the reason why it appears to be more addicting than morphine. In the U.S.A. and many other countries its use for medical purposes is illegal, although this seems to have contributed little to solving the problem of addiction.

Levorphanol and dextromoramide are well absorbed by mouth, and are valuable in the management of chronic pain in terminal disease. Levorphanol is the longer-acting of the two.

Phenazocine is more potent than morphine, but in equianalgesic doses it possibly produces less sedation, vomiting and hypotension than morphine. Its respiratory depressant effect is greater, and it is not the drug of choice in obstetrics or in patients with chest disease. Unlike morphine, it does not affect the sphincter of Oddi.

Pentazocine seems to have a low addiction potential, and for this reason is not controlled by the Misuse of Drugs Act. A withdrawal syndrome occurs, but is mild compared with morphine withdrawal. Pentazocine was developed originally as a narcotic antagonist and like them it can cause hallucinations, bad dreams and thought disturbances, but not as often. Nevertheless the frequency with which they occur is a major disadvantage, and may, in part, account for the low addiction potential of the drug. It is not the drug of choice in myocardial infarction, for it increases pulmonary and systemic blood pressures and left ventricular work. It has a potency somewhere between codeine and morphine. It has an unpredictable effect orally and is usually given parenterally.

Papaveretum is a mixture of purified opium alkaloids in proportions which occur naturally. Almost 50 per cent is morphine, so 20 mg of papaveretum is approximately equivalent to 10 mg of morphine in terms of its analgesic effects. It has no particular advantages.

(b) Pethidine group, including pethidine and phenoperidine, but the latter drug has been used mainly for neuroleptanalgesia. They are synthetic, and although their structures bear only slight resemblance to that of morphine they have many actions in common with this drug. Pethidine is less potent than morphine, but in equianalgesic doses it produces less constipation, nausea and vomiting. Although it was initially developed as a spasmolytic drug, and it has been claimed to have atropine-like effects when used as an analgesic, these properties are weak or non-existent, and it is not superior to morphine for pain of visceral origin. It does not affect the pupil, and does not reduce cough. It has a shorter duration of action than morphine and may be disappointing orally. It produces less sedation and euphoria, but addiction occurs readily.

Phenoperidine is more potent than morphine in its analgesic and respiratory depressant effects. It produces little sedation, but when given with the butyrophenone, droperidol, it produces the twilight state of neuroleptanalgesia.

(c) Methadone group, including methadone and dipipanone. These are synthetic heptanones, only remotely related chemically to morphine. They produce much less sedation, euphoria, respiratory depression and miosis. Methadone is useful for controlling morphine withdrawal symptoms in addicts undergoing treatment. Both drugs are satisfactorily absorbed orally, and are used in the management of chronic pain in terminal disease. Dextropropoxyphene is a mild analgesic related structurally to methadone, and has become popular for treating mild pain. Alone, its effects are significantly inferior to those of aspirin, but in combination with aspirin or paracetamol (Distalgesic contains the latter) it is a useful, although expensive, analgesic. Concern is being expressed, however, over its ability to produce addiction, and over-dosage can be difficult to manage because the patient's state may fluctuate widely, showing features of stimulation and depression in which respiratory depression can be predominant. Furthermore, interaction with alcohol can be hazardous.

(d) Codeine group, including the naturally occurring alkaloid codeine, the semisynthetic dihydrocodeine and pholcodine. Codeine is a weak analgesic to which dependence rarely occurs. It is used in somatic pain, as a cough suppressant and as an antidiarrhoeal (as codeine phosphate). A variety of commercial preparations contain a low dose of codeine in combination with aspirin or paracetamol. Full analgesic doses of codeine produce too much constipation for long term treatment to be practical. Dihydrocodeine has an analgesic potency somewhere between codeine and morphine. Orally it is often more effective than pethidine, but like codeine it constipates and can produce unpleasant dizziness. Pholcodine is used only as an antitussive.

Narcotic antagonists
Nalorphine, levallorphan and naloxone are structurally related to morphine but have only weak analgesic properties. They can counteract the respiratory depressant effects of most narcotic drugs, and are invaluable as specific anatagonists in narcotic overdosage. Naloxone is the drug of choice because it lacks respiratory depressant properties, whereas nalorphine and levallorphan will produce severe depression if given inadvertently to a patient who has overdosed with hypnotic drugs rather than opiates. Nalorphine, but not levallorphan, can induce a severe withdrawal syndrome in a narcotic addict. In a belief that levallorphan antagonizes the respiratory depressant but not the analgesic effect of pethidine, these two compounds have been combined as 'Pethilorfan' for obstetric analgesia in an attempt to prevent depression of breathing in the newborn while providing good analgesia in the mother. In practice, this preparation seems no better in this respect than pethidine alone.

Narcotic antagonists have analgesic effects of their own, but they can cause hallucinations and unpleasant affective and thought disturbances if given in sufficient dosage to produce useful analgesia.

Buprenorphine is an agonist/antagonist which is used as a longacting analgesic in place of morphine. It has minimal effects on the cardiovascular system, a relatively low addiction potential, and is incompletely reversed by naloxone.

Treatment of acute pain
Parental preparations are required for treating acute pain. If they are injected subcutaneously or intramuscularly into a shocked patient, they are poorly absorbed from vasoconstricted tissues. Under these circumstances they should be injected slowly intravenously until effective analgesia has been achieved. This method is also useful for determining the dose of drug required to produce

pain relief with subsequent intramuscular maintenance therapy.

The choice of drug depends largely upon the severity of the pain. Morphine and heroin are the most effective in severe pain, but phenazocine is a useful alternative. Their various advantages and disadvantages have been considered above. Pethidine and pentazocine are unable to produce analgesia equivalent to that of morphine, however large the dose, and are therefore suitable only for milder pain. Pethidine has been the most popular analgesic in obstetrics for a number of years because it depresses the respiratory centre of the newborn less than morphine and is shorter in its duration of action. Recent trials have suggested that pentazocine may be as satisfactory as pethidine for this purpose. Dihydrocodeine is satisfactory in mild pain, but it constipates on repeated dosage.

Acute pain is often accompanied by anxiety, which can in turn make the pain worse. Morphine and heroin are particularly useful in this circumstance, for they produce marked sedation and euphoria which contribute substantially to the resulting analgesia. It is unnecessary to administer a tranquillizer or sedative at the same time. Indeed, it is a hazardous practice to inject an opiate and another central depressant drug simulatenously, for the respiratory depressant effect of the opiate may be potentiated to an extent where repiratory arrest occurs.

Powerful narcotic drugs should be prescribed for only a few days for postoperative pain and other acutely painful conditions, because dependence becomes a risk if treatment is continued longer. A withdrawal syndrome is usually seen when morphine is stopped after about 1 to 2 weeks of continuous use.

Treatment of chronic pain

In the management of pain accompanying terminal disease, oral treatment is desirable where possible. An aqueous solution of morphine or diamorphine given orally is satisfactory as a first choice of narcotic analgesic. The object of treatment should be to prevent pain rather than to suppress it each time it returns. The narcotic should be given four-hourly in a dose which has been titrated to free the patient of pain. Tolerance and addiction are seldom a problem. Drowsiness usually passes within a few days, and respiratory depression is rarely troublesome. Constipation is frequent and may require a regular laxative.

As alternatives to morphine, drugs of moderate strength such as papaveretum or dipipanone can be used. A stronger narcotic may become necessary, when levorphanol, dextromoramide or phenazocine are suitable. Methadone is cumulative and difficult to manage, and pethidine and pentazocine have too short a duration of action and are poorly effective.

Parenteral analgesics may be necessary when intractable nausea and vomiting do not respond to anti-emetics. Diamorphine is best because it is more soluble than morphine and a smaller volume can be injected.

Phenothiazines have been used to potentiate the analgesic action of opiates, although the effectiveness of this remains to be proven. However, phenothiazines will control nausea and vomiting produced either by the disease or by the opiate. Mixtures of cocaine, heroin and alcohol have been used for many years, but there is no evidence that cocaine reduces drowsiness or enhances mood, and some patients dislike the alcohol.

Non-analgesic uses
Because of their ability to produce sedation and euphoria opiates have long been used for premedication. Other marginal benefits result from their use in this situation, including a lessening of mucus and saliva production, and a reduced incidence of cardiac and respiratory irregularities. Respiratory depression, nausea, vomiting and constipation are drawbacks, however.

Similarly, morphine has been used widely for sedating patients with haematemesis, but as these patients are often hypovolaemic and shocked intramuscular injections can be poorly absorbed.

The dyspnoea produced by pulmonary oedema (e.g. paroxysmal nocturnal dyspnoea) is greatly reduced by morphine, and improved ventilation assists reabsorption of the fluid from the alveoli. But it is critical to distinguish between the dyspnoea of pulmonary oedema and that of status asthmaticus, for morphine may precipitate respiratory failure in the latter condition. Fortunately, the development of potent diuretic drugs such as frusemide, bumetanide and ethacrynic acid have made the administration of morphine unnecessary in pulmonary oedema, and therefore the danger resulting from misdiagnosis is eliminated.

Contraindications
Narcotic analgesics should never be used in the following conditions:

    (a) Respiratory disease. Respiratory failure can result.

    (b) Liver disease. Hepatic encephalopathy may ensue.

    (c) Hypothyroidism, hypopituitarism or Addison's disease. Coma may be precipitated.

    (d) Raised intracranial tension. Coma may be precipitated.

(e) Head injury. Valuable pupil signs may be lost.

Patients receiving a MAOI should not be given a narcotic analgesic, for the effects of the analgesic can be greatly exaggerated, producing excitation, rigidity, coma, hyperpyrexia and changes in blood pressure, more commonly hypotension.

Narcotic dependence

Dependence can be induced in any subject given a narcotic in sufficient dosage for a sufficient time, but addiction, with all its physical, psychological and social implications, occurs only in those who need an escape from reality. A discussion of these problems is beyond the scope of this book.

Withdrawal of morphine from an addict produces a withdrawal syndrome, comprising restlessness, anxiety, yawning, sweating and lacrimation. After about 24 hours cramps, muscle twitching, vomiting and diarrhoea begin, and reach a peak at 48 to 72 hours. Insomnia and hallucinations occur. The syndrome settles after 5 to 10 days. Injection of an opiate antagonist can precipitate this syndrome in an addict, and it has been used as a diagnostic test, but it is dangerous unless performed by one experienced in this field. Cross-dependence between many different opiates occurs, and this is utilized in controlling morphine or heroin withdrawal symptoms with methadone.

8

Drugs on the heart

The effects of drugs acting on the heart can be classified as follows:

(a) *Effects on the myocardium.* Changes in the force of contraction of the myocardium are called *inotropic* effects, while changes in the heart rate are called *chronotropic* effects. Drugs which increase the force of contraction or heart rate by direct effect on the myocardium are said to have positive inotropic or chronotropic actions while those which reduce the force of contraction or slow the heart directly have negative intropic or chronotropic effects.

(b) *Effects on the conducting tissue*, particularly on the atrioventricular node and the bundle of His. Drugs may increase or decrease the rate of conduction, directly or indirectly.

(c) *Effects on autonomic control.* In general terms the activity of the heart is stimulated by sympathetic nervous activity and inhibited by vagal parasympathetic activity.

DRUGS WITH POSITIVE INOTROPIC ACTIVITY

Digitalis and related glycosides

These drugs are widely distributed in nature being found in many different plants including the foxglove, squill, Christmas rose, lily of the valley, yellow oleander and wallflower. Official digitalis is the dried leaf of the common foxglove *Digitalis purpurea*, but other varieties of foxglove such as *Digitalis lanata* also contain digitalis glycosides which are extracted commercially. The chief of these is lanatoside C, from which digoxin is derived by hydrolysis. Ouabain is derived from *Strophanthus gratus*. The active constituents of these plant derivatives are *glycosides*, each glycoside being a combination of an *aglycone* or *genin* with sugar molecules. The pharmacological activity resides in the aglycone, while the sugar molecules are thought to influence water solubility and cell penetration.

Actions on the heart

(a) *Myocardium.* The digitalis glycosides have a positive inotropic action on the heart, increasing the systolic force of contraction and so achieving more complete ventricular emptying. These effects are not easily seen in the normal heart because of homeostatic adjustments in the circulatory system. In the failing heart, however, the increased contractile force increases cardiac output and reduces the end-diastolic pressure of the ventricle. The mechanism of this inotropic action is not clear, but probably involves several different factors including a direct effect on the mechanical efficiency of the contractile protein and a change in distribution of calcium and potassium ions in the myocardial cells and extracellular fluid. The increased cardiac work is accomplished without a commensurate increase in oxygen consumption, that is, myocardial efficiency is increased.

While exerting its positive inotropic effect on the myocardium, digitalis also increases its excitability, which results in the production of ectopic beats when excessive doses are administered.

(b) *Conducting tissue.* Conduction in the bundle of His is depressed, with increase in atrioventricular conduction time and lengthening of the $P-R$ interval on the electrocardiogram.

(c) *Autonomic control.* Digitalis increases vagal tone on the heart resulting in slowing of the sinoatrial nodal rate, and further depression of conduction in the bundle of His. This action may be abolished by atropine.

Electrocardiographic changes

Treatment with digitalis produces changes in the electrocardiogram. The earliest effect is depression of the horizontal $S-T$ segment, followed by a biphasic T wave. Ultimately the T wave becomes entirely inverted leading steeply from the depressed $S-T$ segment. The $P-R$ interval may be prolonged due to slowing of atrioventricular conduction, and the $Q-T$ portion shortened due to reduction in duration of ventricular systole.

Other actions

(a) *Central nervous system.* Digitalis has a direct action on the central nervous system, producing vomiting and convulsions in animals and visual disturbances, vertigo, delerium and rarely peripheral neuropathy in man. These central nervous disturbances may precede clinical evidence of cardiac toxicity and are valuable warning signs.

(b) *Kidney.* See Chapter 10.

(c) *Endocrine effects.* The digitalis glycosides are steroid derivatives and this may account for rare endocrine disturbances that they may produce including gynaecomastia and changes in vaginal epithelium indicating some oestrogen-like activity.

Absorption and excretion

The digitalis glycosides vary markedly in their rate of absorption from the gastrointestinal tract. Ouabain is so erratically absorbed that its use is best limited to parenteral administration. Digoxin is the most widely used glycoside and is absorbed rapidly from the gut. It may also be administered intravenously to achieve a more rapid therapeutic effect. Different tablet preparations of digoxin may have differing biological availability even though they all conform to recognized standards of disintegration, and it is important to confirm equivalence of availability before changing the commercial source of digoxin preparations in the treatment of individual patients. The elimination of the digitalis glycosides is slow, varying in rate from one to another, and giving rise to a marked cumulative action (Table 10). Digoxin is eliminated largely by urinary excretion.

Table 10.

Plant source	Glycoside	After single intravenous dose		
		Action begins	Maximal	Action gone
Digitalis purpurea (leaf)	Digitoxin	30 min	4–12 hours	2 weeks
	Gitoxin Gitalin	Seldom used therapeutically		
Digitalis lanata (leaf)	Digitoxin Gitoxin			
	Digoxin	10 min	1–5 hours	2–6 days
Strophanthus gratus (seed)	Ouabain	10 min	½–1 hour	1–3 days

Although digitalizing regimes are described in most medical textbooks it is probably wise to avoid routine dose schedules. There are several factors which modify response to digitalis including age, very young and very old patients being particularly sensitive to its action, and electrolyte imbalance. Hypokalaemia, in particular, potentiates its therapeutic action and may precipitate intoxication. These factors must be considered in any patient, therefore, together with previous treatment with digitalis, diuretics and other drugs which have actions on the heart. When its therapeutic effect is needed rapidly but not urgently digoxin is the preparation of choice. If the patient is vomiting or unable to take it by mouth it may be given intravenously. Ouabain is probably best reserved for very urgent situations when its therapeutic effects appear quickly and reach a maximum within 30 minutes of intravenous injection. Other digitalis glycosides are best reserved for patients who are intolerant of digoxin. The powdered leaf of digitalis is a crude mixture of glycosides and is assayed biologically. It is, therefore, more difficult to ensure an accurate and predictable dose with the leaf than with a single pure glycoside such as digoxin and it should not be considered for routine use.

A radioimmunoassay method is available for determination of plasma level of digoxin after oral therapeutic doses. In the adult, therapeutic plasma concentrations lie between 1·3 and 3·2 nmol/l (1 to 2·5 ng/ml), higher levels being associated with increasing incidence of toxic effects.

Therapeutic indications

(*a*) *Atrial fibrillation*. In this condition the ventricles respond irregularly to bombardment of impulses from the fibrillating atria. Because of the direct and indirect effects of digitalis on conduction time in the Bundle of His, the ventricular rate is slowed and the beats become more regular in strength and time. Longer diastolic filling time allows increased ventricular filling and therefore a greater stroke volume and cardiac output.

(*b*) *Congestive cardiac failure*. Although digitalis is widely used in the treatment of cardiac failure in patients in sinus rhythm, there is considerable uncertainty about its true value. Its positive inotropic effect appears to be relatively short lived and its beneficial action has to be weighed against its important and common adverse effects. It may be preferable to withold digitalis in such patients until aggressive treatment with diuretics, aminophylline and vasodilators (p. 49) has been attempted. Digitalis is certainly indicated, however, in patients whose cardiac failure is associated with atrial fibrillation. When there is frank myocardial disease as in myocarditis and cardiomyopathies of various types, the response to digitalis may be poor.

(*c*) *Atrial flutter*. Treatment with digitalis may lead to conversion either to sinus rhythm or atrial fibrillation with good control of the ventricular rate. When flutter persists the ventricular rate is usually slowed as the result of slower atrioventricular conduction.

(*d*) *Other dysrhythmias*. Frequent episodes of paroxysmal atrial or nodal tachycardia which are not themselves due to digitalis may require treatment with digitalis when other methods of treatment such as carotid sinus stimulation or sedation have failed.

Toxicity

Dose-independent hypersensitivity reactions to digitalis such as urticaria and thrombocytopenia are rare. Digitalis intoxication, however, is a relatively common condition and reports of its frequency in patients receiving the drug vary from 6 to 22 per cent. It is dose-dependent and manifests itself in many ways.

(*a*) *Gastrointestinal symptoms*. Anorexia, nausea and vomiting are common. Abdominal pain and alterations in bowel habit are less frequently seen.

(*b*) *Neurological symptoms*. Headache, fatigue, insomnia, confusion, depression and vertigo are common. Neuralgias, particularly trigeminal, convulsions, paraesthesiae, delirium and psychosis may also occur.

(*c*) *Visual disturbances*. Abnormalities of colour vision with coloured haloes are common. Shimmering vision, scotomata, micropsia and amblyopia occur rarely.

(*d*) *Cardiac manifestations*. Digitalis overdosage may lead to an impairment of cardiac function with precipation or aggravation of congestive cardiac failure. All known types of dysrhythmia have been described in digitalis intoxication, the most common being ventricular ectopic beats which at first are occasional but then progress to 'coupling' with an ectopic beat following closely on a normally generated contraction. If the dose of digitalis is not reduced or discontinued at this stage ventricular tachycardia may follow, and finally ventricular fibrillation. Less commonly atrial dysrhythmias may occur, particularly atrial tachycardia and this may be associated with the development of partial atrioventricular block and an irregular ventricular response. Transient or permanent atrial fibrillation may be induced by digitalis.

Digitalis intoxication is treated by:

(1) Withdrawal of the drug or reduction in its dose.

(2) Administration of potassium. Hypokalaemia, particularly following diuretic therapy, often precipitates digitalis intoxication, and may be corrected by administering potassium orally or intravenously. The latter route should only be used when absolutely necessary, and with great caution, and with continuous electrocardiographic monitoring to prevent toxic signs of hyperkalaemia or cardiac dysrhythmias. Frequent determination of serum potassium should be made.

(3) Antidysrhythmic drugs. Phenytoin and lignocaine are particularly useful.

Glucagon

Glucagon is a polypeptide hormone produced by the α-cells of the pancreatic islets. It has marked hyperglycaemic properties, and in addition has been shown to release insulin, growth hormone, thyroid hormones, calcitonin, parathormone and catecholamines from their respective endocrine glands. It increases the force of cardiac contraction by increasing myocardial adenyl cyclase activity without stimulating the β-adrenoceptor, and therefore its action is not blocked by a β-receptor antagonist. This provides evidence for there being at least two myocardial adenyl cyclase systems. However, its maximal inotropic action is relatively weak and in heart failure it is even weaker. Furthermore, nausea and vomiting occur relatively frequently with its use and are dose related. It has been used in shocked patients who have been given large doses of β-receptor blocking drugs, but as these are competitive antagonists their effects can usually be overcome by appropriate doses of β-receptor agonists.

β-Adrenoceptor agonists

Normal myocardial contractility and function are dependent on sympathetic drive. In congestive cardiac failure the myocardium becomes depleted of noradrenaline. Chronic administration of anti-hypertensive drugs such as reserpine and α-methyldopa which deplete myocardial noradrenaline stores may lead to further cardiac decompensation. With such depletion, reflex sympathetic activity can no longer produce the increased performance required to compensate for mycardial failure. However, if catecholamines with predominant β-receptor stimulating activity such as isoprenaline, salbutamol or dobutamine (p. 40) are given, sympathetic drive may be increased and function improved.

Continuous intravenous infusion of isoprenaline has been shown to increase cardiac output and reduce left ventricular end-diastolic pressure in various forms of heart disease including mitral stenosis and insufficiency, aortic regurgitation and various cardiomyopathies. They are particularly helpful in treating bradycardia or hypotension when these complicate congestive failure or other low-output states, but are of little value in severe coronary artery disease and aortic stenosis. In addition to their inotropic action, however, they possesses marked chronotropic effects and this produces the risk of cardiac dysrhythmias. Continuous monitoring of heart rate and rhythm is, therefore, necessary.

Although electrical pacing is now the treatment of choice in heart block and Stokes–Adams attacks, the positive chronotropic effect of β-agonists is still exploited in the management of some cases. A sustained-release preparation of isoprenaline, 'Saventrine', is sometimes used in long-term management.

Dopamine has less α-receptor agonist activity than noradrenaline and produces less tachycardia than isoprenaline. It has similar inotropic activity, however, and is of value in some patients with cardiogenic shock. In lower doses it dilates renal, mesenteric, coronary and pulmonary vessels, probably by stimulating specific dopamine receptors, but higher doses produce dysrrhythmias and α-adrenoceptor mediated vasoconstriction.

Xanthine drugs. See pages 40 and 145.

ANTIDYSRHYTHMIC DRUGS

Cardiac dysrhythmias arise from ectopic foci in the atria or ventricles, which develop when the sino-atrial node is suppressed or when other conducting tissues or parts of the myocardium depolarize more rapidly. There are a large number of factors which favour rapid depolarization including ischaemia and other forms of injury to the myocardium, digitalis, catecholamines, atropine, hypocalcaemia and respiratory acidosis.

Drugs which suppress dysrhythmias may be divided into three groups:

(1) Membrane stabilizing drugs.
(2) Adrenergic neurone and receptor blocking drugs.
(3) Calcium antagonists.

Membrane stabilizing drugs
These drugs share the common property of raising the threshold of the myocardium to stimulation by direct membrane stabilizing action.

Quinidine. Quinidine, a stereoisomer of quinine, has myocardial depressant and local anaesthetic activity. A comparison of its effects with digitalis on the myocardium, conducting tissue and autonomic control is shown in Table 11.

Quinidine depresses myocardial contractility and conduction, having a direct action on ion transport across the cell membrane. Therefore, although like digitalis it slows the rate of atrioventricu-

Table 11

	Myocardial excitability	Myocardial contractility	A-V conduction rate	Vagal tone
Digitalis	Increased	Increased	Slowed	Increased
Quinidine	Decreased	Decreased	Slowed	Reduced

lar conduction, it does not improve myocardial contractility but depresses it and may lead to a reduction in cardiac output.

Quinidine is used (1) prophylactically to prevent recurrent paroxysmal dysrhythmias such as atrial fibrillation or flutter, and atrial or ventricular ectopic beats, and (2) therapeutically in paroxysmal atrial or ventricular tachycardias, atrial flutter or in attempted conversion of atrial fibrillation to sinus rhythm. Electrical cardioversion has now largely supplanted its use in the latter indication, however.

Quinidine is contraindicated in partial and complete heart block, and in digitalis-induced dysrhythmias. Its effects are cumulative, persisting for 6 to 8 hours, and a patient receiving it therapeutically should be under close observation for evidence of toxicity. Among its toxic manifestations are dose-independent hypersensitivity reactions including urticaria and signs of anaphylaxis, and purpura due to thrombocytopenia. Dose-dependent effects include vertigo, tinnitus, deafness and blurred vision, mental confusion, nausea, vomiting, diarrhoea, and disorders of cardiac rhythm including ectopic beats, atrioventricular block, ventricular fibrillation and the cardiac arrest. These cardiac effects are usually preceded by electrocardiographic evidence of toxicity characterized by a prolongation of the *QRS* interval to 0·12 seconds or more.

Procainamide. Procainamide has similar pharmacological properties to procaine but is destroyed less rapidly and so exerts a more prolonged action. Its central stimulant action is also said to be less than that of procaine. It is used in the treatment of atrial and ventricular ectopic beats and dysrhythmias, and may be used prophylactically following myocardial infarction to prevent the development of major dysrhythmias. It has a narrow therapeutic ratio, however, and it is desirable to monitor drug plasma levels whenever possible. The effective plasma concentration appears to be 5 to 6 μg per ml, lower levels giving incomplete protection, and concentrations above 7 μg per ml producing hypotension and electrocardiographic evidence of heart block. Sustained plasma concentrations are best achieved by using slow-release preparations, as the drug has a short elimination half-life. Treatment with procainamide is contraindicated in the presence of atrioventricular or intraventricular block.

Adverse effects of procainamide include cardiac dysrhythmias, hypotension, mental depression and hallucinations. An important hypersensitivity reaction consists of a syndrome which at first resembles early rheumatoid arthritis but develops into a condition indistinguishable from disseminated lupus erythematosus if procainamide treatment is continued. Procainamide is subject to acetylation and there is evidence that slow acetylators develop antibodies and the lupus syndrome earlier and with lower total cumulative doses than rapid acetylators (p. 21).

Lignocaine. Lignocaine, like quinidine and procainamide, is a local anaesthetic agent which is an effective antidysrrhythmic drug. It is particularly useful in the treatment of ventricular dysrhythmias associated with myocardial infarction and digitalis overdosage. It is ineffective in supraventricular dysrhythmias. Its systemic bioavailability after oral administration is poor because of extensive hepatic extraction and metabolism, and it is therefore usually administered by intravenous injection or infusion. Like procainamide its therapeutic ratio is small, and optimum serum levels lie between 1·5 and 3·0 μg/ml. Adverse effects include hypotension, central nervous depression and convulsions. It is contraindicated in the presence of atrioventricular or intraventricular block. Cardiac failure and liver dysfunction can lead to reduced clearance and accumulation of lignocaine.

Disopyramide. Disopyramide resembles quinidine in that it prolongs the refractory period of the A-V node, slows conduction in the bundle of His and Purkinje fibre system, and reduces atrial and ventricular excitability. Its uses are similar to those of quinidine, but it is less toxic, its principle adverse effects being depression of cardiac contractility and anticholinergic actions. It can be administered orally and parenterally, and has proved of special value in the prophylaxis of ventricular dysrhythmias after myocardial infarction, in which the therapeutic range appears to be between 2 and 4 μg/ml. Because of its myocardial depressant action, it should be used with caution in patients with impaired cardiac contractility. Its anticholinergic adverse effects are relatively common and include urinary retention, blurred vision and dry mouth. It should be used with caution in patients at risk of bladder neck obstruction or glaucoma.

Mexiletine. Mexilentine is the most recently introduced antidysrhythmic agent which, while still undergoing assessment, appears to be effective orally and parenterally in suppressing ventricular dysrhythmias, particularly following myocardial infarction. Its principle adverse effects include hypotension, nausea, vomiting, dysphoria, and cerebellar signs of nystagmus and ataxia.

Phenytoin. Phenytoin is an anticonvulsant drug with membrane-stabilizing properties which is particularly effective in suppressing digitalis-induced supraventricular and ventricular dysrhythmias, although it is also useful in patients with postmyocardial infarction dysrhythmias. The critical plasma level for its optimum effect appears to lie between 10 and 18 μg per ml. Its adverse effects after prolonged use are dealt with elsewhere (Chapter 6), but its intravenous administration for antidysrhythmic purposes carries the particular risks of hypotension, heart block and cardiac and respiratory arrest.

Adrenergic neurone and receptor blocking drugs
Drugs which block the adrenergic neurone or cardiac receptors would be expected to reduce the incidence of dysrhythmias which are associated with sympathetic activity, for example those occurring during induction of anaesthesia with cyclopropane or halothane.

Adrenergic neurone blocking drugs, particularly bretylium, afford significant protection against digitalis-induced dysrhythmias in animals, without possessing direct membrane-stabilizing effects. They are unsuitable for routine antidysrhythmic treatment, however, because of their associated hypotensive action.

It is uncertain whether α-adrenergic receptor blockade is associated with antidysrhythmic activity. Indoramin, an α-receptor blocking drug, possesses antidysrhythmic properties, but this may be due to its membrane-stabilizing activity which is seen at higher plasma concentrations than its α-receptor blocking effects.

β-Receptor blockade prevents dysrhythmias which are associated with sympathetic overactivity, or with increased circulating catecholamines. It is, therefore, indicated in the treatment of patients with phaeochromocytoma. β-Blocking drugs such as propranolol, however, also protect against digitalis-induced dysrhythmias, and as propranolol also possesses local anaesthetic and membrane-stabilizing properties it has been suggested that these, rather than β-blockade, account for its antidysrhythmic activity. However, the dextro-isomer of propranolol which is equipotent with the laevo form in terms of membrane stabilization but possesses only about 1 per cent of its β-receptor blocking activity is markedly less effective in protection against digitalis-induced dysrhythmias in animals. Similarly, the plasma levels of racemic propranolol associated with suppression of ventricular ectopic beats are in the same range as those causing β-adrenergic blockade, and are less than 1 per cent of those required *in vitro* to demonstrate local anaesthetic or membrane stabilizing effects on isolated human myocardial tissue. It appears, therefore, that the antidysrhythmic effect of propranolol and other β-adrenergic receptor blocking drugs is due primarily to their β-blocking action rather than to other properties such as membrane stabilization which they demonstrate in higher concentrations.

Calcium antagonists

These drugs, which are still being assessed clinically, appear to block calcium influx across myocardial cell membranes and this may be responsible for their observed antidysrhythmic properties.

Verapamil is a derivitive of papaverine which appears to be effective in the control and prevention of atrial dysrhythmias and is also used in the prophylaxis of angina pectoris. Adverse effects include hypotension, cardiac failure, bradycardia and cardiac arrest, and these are particularly likely to occur in patients also receiving β-adrenoceptor blocking drugs. Verapamil should not, therefore, be administered to patients who are being treated with these drugs.

Nifedipine is a powerful calcium antagonist which not only influences myocardial function but also causes peripheral vasodilatation. It is being assessed primarily in the management of angina pectoris (p. 134).

CORONARY ARTERIES

Coronary artery tone depends on (a) the intrinsic tone of the vessel wall, (b) the metabolic state of the myocardium and (c) autonomic nervous activity. Studies of the pharmacology of the coronary arteries are difficult because it is not easy to keep any two of these variables constant to allow controlled change of the third. As with blood vessels elsewhere in the body, an accumulation of metabolites in the cardiac muscle is a potent stimulus to vasodilatation. Furthermore, coronary flow depends on aortic blood pressure, and a reduction in this is followed by a fall in flow. Another problem is that stimulation of autonomic nervous activity causes not only changes in aortic pressure and coronary tone but also changes the rate and force of the contracting cardiac muscle, which then influences coronary vascular resistance passively.

There appears to be no direct vagal innervation of the coronary arteries. Acetylcholine and other cholinergic drugs injected intravenously may cause coronary dilatation, but because of the simultaneous fall in aortic pressure which they produce, coronary flow may actually fall.

The coronary arteries are under sympathetic nervous control, being predominantly vasodilator. Adrenaline and noradrenaline produce an initial constriction when injected directly into the coronary vessels, but this is followed by dilatation which is probably due to direct effects on adrenergic receptors in the vessel walls and also, to a smaller extent, to changes in myocardial metabolic processes. After β-receptor blockade with propranolol the vasodilator effects of adrenaline and noradrenaline disappear and are replaced by prolonged constriction. This suggests that coronary vessels possess constrictor α-adrenergic receptors and dilator β-receptors.

Drugs in angina pectoris
(a) Nitrites and organic nitrates. Members of this group of vasodilator drugs remain the most effective agents available for the treatment of angina pectoris. They include the nitrites sodium nitrite and amyl nitrite, and the organic nitrates glyceryl trinitrate, erythrityl tetranitrate, pentaerythritol tetranitrate and isosorbide dinitrate. Although they produce dilatation of normal coronary arteries, it is unlikely that they have significant effects on the calcified and atheromatous vessels which are present in patients with ischaemic heart disease. In any case, the accumulation of myocardial metabolites in an anginal attack is probably a better stimulus to vasodilatation than drug treatment. Their principal mechanism of action is general systemic arterial dilatation throughout the body, reducing blood pressure, and cardiac work. There is, therefore, a reduction in the myocardial oxygen requirement, and this, rather than an increase in coronary flow, is responsible for their effectiveness in angina. There are some relatively minor regional differences in action of various compounds. For example, amyl nitrite causes reflex venoconstriction while glyceryl trinitrate dilates both the arteriolar and venous beds of the human forearm.

The general arterial dilatation which these drugs produce is responsible for the flushing, throbbing headache, transient dizziness and reflex tachycardia which follow their administration.

Amyl nitrite is a volatile liquid, administered in thin glass capsules wrapped in cloth which are broken and inhaled. It acts within a few seconds, and its effects last for about 10 minutes.

Glyceryl trinitrate (nitroglycerine) is administered as a tablet for sublingual application, the effects being seen within 2 minutes and lasting for up to 20 or 30 minutes. As well as relieving the pain of an acute attack, it may be used prophylactically before physical exertion or mental stress which would be expected to produce an anginal attack.

Isosorbide dinitrate, erythrityl tetranitrate and pentaerythritol tetranitrate are more stable compounds which are administered orally 3 or 4 times daily for prophylaxis of angina, but their therapeutic usefulness has not been established. Isosorbide dinitrate is being increasingly but cautiously used to reduce preload in patients with intractable heart failure unresponsive to diuretic therapy (p. 125), by producing generalised venodilatation and reduced venous return.

The principal toxic effect of these compounds is the production of methaemoglobinaemia due to oxidation of haemoglobin, but this is seldom seen in therapeutic doses. When over 10 per cent of haemoglobin is oxidized to methaemoglobin, the patient's skin may have a slaty-blue appearance due to the characteristic chocolate colour of methaemoglobin.

(b) β -Adrenergic receptor blocking drugs. See Chapter 5.

(c) Other drugs. Verapamil and nifedipine are calcium antagonists that reduce the number and severity of anginal attacks in patients with ischaemic heart disease (p. 132). Their anti-anginal mechanism of action is uncertain.

Prenylamine depletes myocardial stores of noradrenaline, but it is less effective than reserpine in this respect, and as reserpine is of little value in angina it is unlikely that this effect is responsible for its anti-anginal action. Its therapeutic effect develops slowly, reduction in frequency of anginal attacks appearing after 10 to 14 days of treatment. Hypotension may appear with prolonged treatment, and the dose of concurrently administered anti-hypertensive drugs may require adjustment.

Dipyridamole is a potent coronary vasodilator in animals and normal human subjects, but its value in the treatment of coronary artery disease is uncertain. It also inhibits adenosine-diphosphate-induced aggregation of platelets, and so reduces platelet stickiness.

Perhexiline reduces the frequency and severity of anginal attacks by an unknown mechanism. It does not appear to be either a β-receptor blocking drug or a peripheral vasodilator in therapeutic doses. However, unwanted effects are common and include abnormalities in liver function tests and peripheral neuropathy.

HYPOCHOLESTEROLAEMIC DRUGS

The association of atherosclerosis and ischaemic heart disease with high blood levels of cholesterol and lipids has led to the introduction of hypocholesterolaemic drugs into the treatment of these conditions. Oestrogens reduce serum cholesterol and lipids but their feminizing and other effects discourage their general use, particularly in male patients. Triparanol was withdrawn from use because of the development of irreversible cataracts and other adverse effects. Nicotinic acid in high doses lowers serum cholesterol but adverse effects such as gastrointestinal disturbances, paraesthesiae, flushing of the skin, rashes, lesions resembling acanthosis nigricans, and hyperuricaemia have discouraged its long-term use.

Clofibrate acts at an early stage in cholesterol biosynthesis, lowering serum cholesterol and triglycerides by about 20 to 40 per cent in the majority of patients, particularly those with raised levels before treatment. It also has other important pharmacological properties including prolongation of the prothrombin time in patients receiving hypoprothrombinaemic drugs, reduction in abnormal platelet stickiness, increase in blood fibrinolytic activity and reduction in blood fibrinogen levels. Although its hypocholesterolaemic action in patients with increased blood lipids may be easily demonstrated, and there is evidence that it may significantly reduce the incidence of non-fatal myocardial infarction, trials have shown that the overall mortality is paradoxically increased. The use of clofibrate in the primary prevention of heart disease is therefore inadvisable. Clofibrate has also been claimed to reduce tissue lipids and produce significant improvement in such conditions as tuberous xanthomatosus and exudative lipaemic retinopathy in diabetic patients. Adverse effects of treatment are uncommon, the most frequent being mild gastrointestinal symptoms. Alopecia, muscle pain and an increased incidence of gall stones and gall bladder disease have also been described.

9

Prostaglandins, platelets and clotting

PROSTAGLANDINS

Prostaglandin was the name originally given to a lipid substance derived from human seminal plasma which contracted smooth muscle. Substances with similar activity were found in seminal fluid from other animals, and in extracts of prostate and vesicular glands. Today the term prostaglandin refers to a large family of closely related long-chain unsaturated fatty acids, all derivatives of prostanoic acid. They are identified by alphabetical and numerical subscripts. Under suitable conditions a large number of tissues and organs can be induced to release prostaglandins into the circulation but their contribution to pharmacological and physiological activity has not yet been fully elucidated. There is, however, increasing evidence for important roles in several processes. Prostaglandins of the E and F groups appear to be associated with various kinds of inflammatory reactions, and it may be that part, at least, of the anti-inflammatory action of drugs such as aspirin, indomethacin and phenylbutazone is due to their inhibitory effects on prostaglandin synthetase, an enzyme intimately concerned in their formation. Some prostaglandins have also been used to induce abortion in early pregnancy, and labour in the last trimester (see p. 179).

It is thought that prostaglandin E maintains the patency of the foetal ductus arteriosus because administration of non-steroidal anti-inflammatory drugs to the mother to inhibit premature labour has resulted in premature closure (p. 180). However, this observation has lead to the use of non-steroidal anti-inflammatory drugs to promote a 'chemical' ligation of patent ductus in neonates. Success has been variable but is greatest in babies less than 14 days old.

Appreciable quantities of prostaglandins are present in brain tissue, and microinjection techniques have shown stimulating and inhibiting actions on neurones in the central nervous system. It may be, therefore, that some of these substances are concerned directly or indirectly with central transmission.

Various prostaglandins have been shown to have vasoconstrictor, vasodilator, bronchoconstrictor and bronchodilator activity. Some prostaglandins of the E type decrease gastric acid production and increase blood flow in the gastric musculature. The gastric side effects of phenylbutazone and indomethacin may be due to inhibition of prostaglandin synthesis by these agents.

Prostacyclin
Prostacyclin (originally called PGI_2) was discovered as recently as

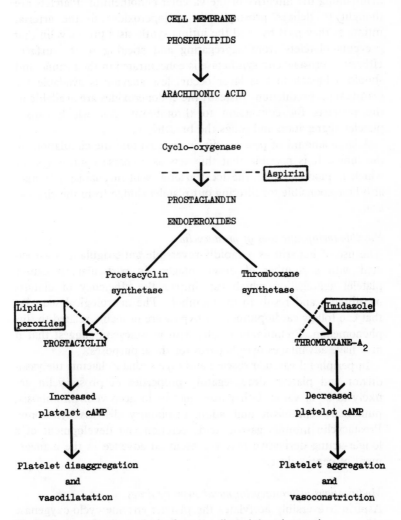

Fig. 14 Pathway for the synthesis of prostacyclin and thromboxane-A_2.

1976. It is synthesised from arachidonic acid in arterial walls (Fig. 14) and it is potent in preventing platelet aggregation, as well as causing vasodilatation. The former effect appears to be mediated by an increase in the concentration of cyclic AMP in platelets.

Arachidonic acid metabolism also leads to the synthesis of thromboxane-A_2 which has opposite effects to prostacyclin. It reduces platelet cyclic AMP, leading to platelet aggregation, and also causes vasoconstriction.

It has been suggested that these substances play a natural role in maintaining the integrity of the vascular endothelium. Platelets are thought to deliver prostaglandin endoperoxides to the arterial intima as they pass by, and the intima synthesises prostacyclin that prevents platelets from aggregating and sticking to its surface. However, prostacyclin synthetase is concentrated in the intima, and should a breach in this layer occur, less enzyme is available for prostacyclin production. Instead, the endoperoxides are available in the platelets for conversion to thromboxane-A_2, which causes platelet aggregation and plugs the breach.

A large amount of prostacyclin is secreted into the circulation by the lungs. It is possible that this acts as a coarse control system which is modulated by the local arterial wall mechanism. It may also be responsible for filtering out platelet sludge from the circulation.

Possible therapeutic uses of prostacyclin

The use of heparin as a rapidly-reversible anticoagulant is associated with a number of disadvantages. In particular, it causes platelet aggregation which can impair the efficiency of dialysis membranes and result in microemboli. The neurological sequelae that can follow cardiopulmonary bypass are probably related to this phenomenon. Preliminary results with prostacyclin suggest that it may have advantages over heparin for these purposes.

In peripheral vascular disease and myocardial ischaemia the vasodilator and platelet deaggregating properties of prostacyclin are likely to be of value. Other uses may be in deep vein thrombosis, pulmonary embolism and adult respiratory distress syndrome. Prostacyclin inhibits gastric acid secretion and development of a longer-acting derivative may represent an advance in the management of peptic ulcer.

Modifications of prostacyclin metabolism by drugs

Aspirin irreversibly acetylates the platelet enzyme cyclo-oxygenase (Fig. 14), thereby preventing the formation of thromboxane A_2. In conventional doses it also reversibly inhibits the same enzyme in the blood vessel wall, and blocks the formation of prostacyclin. In terms of thrombotic disease, these two effects oppose each other because thromboxane A_2 is pro-aggregatory while prostacyclin is deaggregatory. However, low doses of aspirin, e.g. 300 mg every third day, appear to spare the vessel wall enzyme, leaving a predominantly deaggregatory effect. So far, clinical trials in the secondary prevention of myocardial infarction (i.e. reducing the morbidity and mortality in patients who have already had a heart attack) have produced contradictory results and further studies are necessary.

Imidazole and other chemicals can selectively inhibit thromboxane synthetase (Fig. 14) and although these do not currently represent a practical form of treatment, future research may produce a compound with clinical application. Lipid peroxides inhibit prostacyclin synthetase, and are found in atheromatous plaques, hyperlipidaemia and vitamin E deficiency. Studies are underway to investigate the therapeutic potential of modifying lipid peroxide activity.

Other inhibitors of platelet aggregation

Dipyridamole, a coronary vasodilator drug (p. 134), also inhibits platelet aggregation induced by adenosine diphosphate. So far, however, clinical trials have failed to show its value in secondary prevention of myocardial infarction.

Sulphinpyrazone, a uricosuric agent, has been shown to have the additional effect of prolonging platelet survival. A major clinical trial of this compound in secondary prevention has shown that it is capable of reducing sudden death rather than reinfarction, and that this was an early effect rather than a continuing one. This result suggests an effect other than on platelet survival, but what this effect might be is unknown.

Anticoagulant drugs

Anticoagulant drugs inhibit the clotting mechanism. Although the latter is an important part of the thrombotic process, it is neither the initiating event nor invariably the dominant factor in thrombosis, and therefore the therapeutic role of anticoagulants in arterial thrombotic disorders is small. However, in venous thrombosis and atrial thromboembolism from mitral valve disease they are of proven value. A thrombus comprises aggregated platelets upon which fibrin deposition subsequently occurs. Conventional anticoagulant drugs do not interfere with the platelet contribution to thrombus formation.

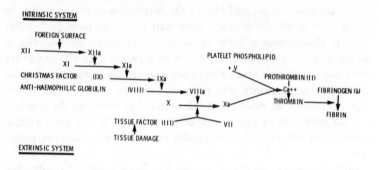

Fig. 15 The clotting mechanism.

Coumarins and indanediones

Coumarins are present in many plants and their anticoagulant effects were discovered on investigation of a haemorrhagic disease in cattle who had fed on mouldy sweet clover. The compounds which are used as anticoagulants are synthetic. They interfere with the hepatic synthesis of prothrombin and factors VII, IX and X, rather than with the clotting mechanism itself (see Fig. 15). Their anticoagulant action begins slowly because the circulating levels of these factors have to fall by normal metabolism before the clotting mechanism is affected. The speed of recovery on stopping an anti-coagulant depends upon the rate of metabolism of the individual drugs.

A number of compounds are available for oral use but the most used are warfarin sodium, phenindione, dicoumarol and nicoumalone. Of these, warfarin sodium and dicoumarol have the longest duration of action, and it takes up to 5 days for the prothrombin time to return to normal after stopping treatment. It is usual to give a loading dose at the start of treatment, followed up by a maintenance dose based on the prothrombin time. The object is to keep this at two to three times the control value, i.e. at 21–36 seconds. If immediate anticoagulation is desirable heparin can be given by intravenous infusion or repeated injections for 48 hours, by which time the oral anticoagulant should be producing an adequate effect.

Sensitivity to oral anticoagulants is increased by liver disease because the production of clotting factors may already be low. Treatment with oral broad-spectrum antibiotics may also increase their anticoagulant effect by reducing intestinal flora. They are highly bound to plasma proteins and can be displaced by other highly bound drugs. Barbiturates can induce their metabolism, producing difficulty with control and, more important, haemorrhagic complications when the patient leaves hospital and stops taking his barbiturate hypnotic.

Haemorrhagic complications demand the administration of vitamin K if serious, but milder bleeding, such as haematuria, will settle if the anticoagulant is discontinued for 24–48 hours until the prothrombin time has returned to an acceptable level, and then recommenced at a slightly lower dose. Phenindione frequently produces adverse effects, including skin rashes, agranulocytosis, fever, jaundice, diarrhoea and steatorrhoea. The other drugs rarely produce adverse effects.

Heparin

Heparin is a mucopolysaccharide which occurs naturally in mast cells. It is prepared commercially from beef lung. Its anticoagulant action is due to its strong negative charge, which produces a high affinity for cationic groups such as those of proteins involved in clotting. It appears to inhibit almost every stage of the clotting sequence, but particularly of activated factor X. It also reduces platelet stickiness, but the relevance of this to its clinical effects is uncertain.

Heparin must be given parenterally, preferably by intravenous infusion or intermittent injection, because it produces painful haematomas when given subcutaneously or intramuscularly. It is usual to give a loading dose of 5000 units followed by infusion of 20 000–30 000 units/24 hours, or alternatively a dose of 10 000 units 6-hourly by injection. Ideally the therapeutic effect should be determined at intervals by estimating the whole blood clotting time or the partial thromboplastin time with kaolin, but in practice this is seldom done as heparin is usually used for a few days at the most and cumulation, as occurs in renal impairment, rarely causes complications during this short time. With more prolonged use, however, haemorrhagic complications are common.

Haemorrhage induced by heparin can be controlled by giving protamine sulphate, which has cationic groups that link with excess heparin. This is seldom necessary, however, as minor haemorrhage is quickly controlled by stopping the drug, which has a duration of action of only 4–6 hours. Heparin should be avoided in patients who have peptic ulcers, ulcerative colitis, piles and other lesions which may be encouraged to bleed. Heparin occasionally produces allergic reactions and thrombocytopenia. Prolonged intramuscular administration of large doses may lead to osteoporosis.

Ancrod

This is an enzyme, extracted from the venom of the Malayan pit viper, which causes intravascular precipitation of fibrinogen. Normal fibrinolytic enzyme systems in reticuloendothelial cells immediately convert the precipitated fibrinogen into soluble products. Obstruction of small vessels does not occur provided the drug is given slowly. Intravenous administration is usual. Although not adequately assessed, it appears to produce spontaneous haemorrhage rarely, and rebound hypercoagulability is not a problem. When the drug is stopped the fibrinogen level returns to normal over the course of several days. Its effects can be reversed by a specific antivenom, but normal clotting will not occur until the fibrinogen level has returned to normal. The occurrence of antibodies has been reported.

Fibrinolytic and antifibrinolytic drugs

A fibrinolytic mechanism is normally responsible for lysing small clots which occur within the vascular system. A plasminogen activator (Fig. 16) is released by the vascular endothelium, and the enzyme which is formed, plasmin, acts on fibrin and fibrinogen to produce soluble derivatives. Plasminogen activators, e.g. streptokinase and urokinase can be administered intravenously and produce the same effect as endogenous activators. In contrast to anticoagulant drugs, fibrinolytic compounds can dissolve established clots, e.g. in deep vein thrombosis and pulmonary embolism, as well as preventing further formation. Although best given by infusion through a catheter whose tip lies close to the clot, this is not often possible and the drug is then given by intravenous infusion. A loading dose is given, followed by a maintenance dose for 48–72 hours.

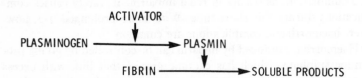

Fig. 16 The fibrinolytic mechanism

Streptokinase is derived from β-haemolytic streptococci. It is highly antigenic and is liable to be inactivated by circulating IgG antibodies from previous streptococcal infections. A loading dose of

250 000 units is sufficient to neutralize the antibody and provide an excess for fibrinolysis. Immediate allergic reactions and pyrexia are so common that it is usual to give prophylactic steroid therapy before the infusion. Urokinase is derived from human kidney-cell cultures or normal urine, and is non-antigenic. It is extremely expensive.

The main risk is of haemorrhage, and an antifibrinolysin (anti-plasmin) such as epsilon aminocaproic acid or tranexamic acid should be available. Antiplasmins are used also in conditions associated with high circulating levels of plasmin, e.g. in concealed or accidental haemorrhage in obstetrics, or following handling of the lungs during surgery. 'Trasylol' is a proprietary preparation with antitrypsin properties as well as being antifibrinolytic, and is used in the treatment of acute pancreatitis, although its value is uncertain.

Indications for use of anticoagulants and fibrinolysins

The indications for use of anticoagulants have been more clearly defined in recent years, with the result that fewer patients are subjected to the risks of haemorrhage when the therapeutic benefit to be gained from treatment is minimal or absent.

(*a*) *Deep vein thrombosis and pulmonary embolism.* Because streptokinase lyses established clots it seems rational to choose this drug when a deep vein thrombosis has been diagnosed. However, the adverse effects of treatment are greater with this drug, and it is preferable to reserve it for more extensive thromboses involving the veins of the thigh and pelvis. For thromboses restricted to the calf, heparin and oral anticoagulants are effective, for clot lysis still occurs by natural mechanisms, even if more slowly. Oral treatment is continued for 6–8 weeks, or long term if recurrent thromboses have occurred.

The realization that deep vein thrombosis occurs in a high percentage of patients undergoing surgery has promoted attempts to prevent clotting. Heparin given immediately before, and for several days after, operation reduces the incidence of thrombosis and subsequent pulmonary embolism. This effect is achieved possibly by reducing platelet stickiness and activating lipoprotein lipase, an enzyme which hydrolyses chylomicra and reduces lipaemia produced by absorption of fats, during which time clotting is normally accelerated. Treatment of high risk patients, e.g. those undergoing gynaecological operations, is important because the incidence of bleeding complications postoperatively is increased.

(*b*) *Mitral valve disease.* When associated with thrombus formation in the left atrium, and microemboli from carotid artery disease.

(c) *Myocardial infarction*. The beneficial effect of anticoagulants immediately after infarction is probably mainly due to the prevention of deep vein thrombosis rather than an effect on the coronary vessels. Men under the age of 55 appear to benefit most. There is some evidence that heparin and streptokinase reduce the mortality and reinfarction rate, but their use cannot be justified because the hazards of anticoagulation weigh heavily against the benefits.

10

Diuretics

A diuretic is a drug which increases the volume of urine produced by the kidney. It may produce its effects in one of two ways:
(a) By increasing renal blood flow and glomerular filtration rate.
(b) By inhibiting the reabsorption of sodium by the renal tubule.

Drug which increase renal blood flow
(a) *Digitalis glycosides*. Cardiac glycosides, such as digoxin, which increase the output of the failing heart and so increase renal perfusion and glomerular filtration, may be said to have diuretic activity. In addition, digoxin has been shown to have a direct action on the renal tubule to inhibit sodium reabsorption, but whether this is important in therapeutic doses is uncertain.

(b) *Xanthines* (see also p. 152). It has long been known that coffee, tea and other related beverages have a diuretic action. This is due to the xanthine drugs caffeine, theobromine and theophylline which they contain. These, together with others such as aminophylline, inhibit the enzyme phosphodiesterase. They increase renal blood flow by increasing the force of cardiac contraction and hence the cardiac output where this is reduced, and by dilating renal medullary blood vessels. They may also directly inhibit sodium reabsorption by the renal tubules. Aminophylline is the most important of this group of drugs in clinical use, and is usually administered by slow intravenous injection.

Drugs which inhibit sodium reabsorption
Fluid retention is usually due to a primary retention of sodium in the body, and the most effective way to reduce excess body water is to increase sodium excretion by the kidneys. It is necessary to induce a state of negative sodium balance in which the quantity of sodium lost by the body is in excess of that taken in.

Sodium reabsorption occurs throughout the length of the renal tubule. The greatest part of the filtered load, between 60 and 70 per cent, is reabsorbed together with water in the proximal part of the tubule. In the ascending limb of the loop of Henle sodium is actively reabsorbed without water, leading to hypertonicity of the surrounding medullary tissue, and hypotonic fluid passes into the distal tubule. Here, under the influence of aldosterone, sodium is exchanged for potassium, and so an increase in the sodium load in the distal part of the distal tubule is associated with increased exchange leading to potassium loss. As the hypotonic filtrate then passes down the collecting tubules through the hypertonic medullary tissue water is reabsorbed under the control of antidiuretic hormone.

(a) *Thiazides.* This group of diuretic agents was developed as the result of a search for more potent carbonic anhydrase inhibitors, although in fact, they owe but little of their action to this effect. Their site of action is uncertain, but probably involves inhibition of sodium reabsorption in the proximal part of the distal tubule. Although they are weaker than the mercurial diuretics (e.g. mersalyl), they have the advantage of being effective after oral administration, and some preparations can be given intravenously. A large number of these compounds are now available including bendrofluazide, chlorothiazide, cyclopenthiazide, hydrocholorothiazide, hydroflumethiazide and polythiazide. Although chemically distinct from the thiazides, chlorthalidone closely resembles them in its pharmacological and adverse effects. It is unlikely that one is superior to another, however, in terms of therapeutic effectiveness or lack of adverse effects, and all show the following features:

(1) Potassium loss. The increased sodium load reaching the distal part of the distal tubule results in an increased exchange of sodium for potassium under the influence of aldosterone. If a marked diuresis occurs with depletion of the blood volume, aldosterone secretion increases leading to an even greater sodium–potassium exchange and potassium loss. Potassium supplements should be given, therefore, to patients receiving regular thiazide treatment.

(2) Hyperglycaemia may occur in patients treated with thiazide drugs, with increased insulin requirements in diabetic patients. The mechanism of this effect is not known.

(3) Hyperuricaemia frequently occurs, with attacks of clinical gout in patients with a previous history of the condition. This is probably due to a reduction in uric acid excretion by the kidney together with contraction of the extracellular fluid volume. Tienilic acid has potentially useful uric-acid excreting and hypouricaemic properties together with diuretic activity. Unfortunately it has been withdrawn from clinical trial because of reports of liver toxicity.

(4) Hypotensive effects (see p. 57).

(b) *Bumetanide and frusemide.* These are related chemically to, but are very much more potent than, the thiazide diuretics. They appear to inhibit sodium reabsorption in the proximal part of the distal tubule, but also have a marked action on the ascending limb of the loop of Henle. They are therefore called 'loop' or 'high-potency' diuretics. For an equivalent degree of diuresis they produce less potassium loss than the thiazides, but when used in larger doses for a powerful diuresis the loss of potassium is considerable and supplementary potassium must be given to patients receiving regular treatment. Excessive sodium and chloride diuresis can lead to severe blood volume depletion, hypotension and uraemia. Like the thiazides they have hyperglycaemic, hyperuricaemic and hypotensive effects. They may be given orally or intravenously, the latter route being particularly appropriate for use in emergencies such as pulmonary oedema.

(c) *Ethacrynic acid.* This drug is of the same order of potency as bumetanide and frusemide, exerting its effect like the latter predominantly on the ascending limb of the loop of Henle and the proximal part of the distal tubule. Its complications and adverse effects are similar with the addition of transient deafness possibly due to interference with the production of perilymph in the inner ear. Its use should be restricted to acute emergencies, in which it may be administered by cautious intravenous injection.

(d) *Spironolactone.* This drug is a synthetic steroid, in structure resembling aldosterone, of which it is a competitive antagonist. It is, therefore, inactive in adrenalectomized patients and its effects are limited in physiological states in which aldosterone secretion is reduced to a minimum. It inhibits the exchange of sodium for potassium ions in the distal part of the distal tubule which is under the control of aldosterone. As the sodium reabsorption here accounts for only a small part of that in the renal tubule as a whole, the diuretic activity of spironolactone is weak. It is most effective in those conditions in which there are high circulating levels of aldosterone, for example, hepatic cirrhosis and the nephrotic syndrome. When given together with diuretics acting at more proximal sites in the nephron, such as the thiazides, it reduces the potassium loss which they produce as well as increasing sodium excretion. It may still be necessary to give potassium supplements, however. Like the thiazides, spironolactone causes a moderate fall in blood pressure by itself, and potentiates the action of other antihypertensive drugs. Toxic effects include headache, nausea and vomiting, and gynaecomastia may occur particularly in men. Hyperkalaemia may occur in patients with renal insufficiency.

(e) *Triamterene*. Triamterene is a pteridine derivative chemically related to inhibitors of folic acid synthesis, but with important diuretic activity. Although it inhibits the exchange of sodium for potassium in the distal tubule, this is independent of aldosterone antagonism, and occurs even in the adrenalectomized animal. Like spironolactone, it is a relatively weak diuretic, but is useful in combination with the thiazides where it potentiates the sodium excreting effect and reduces potassium loss. It is especially useful in those conditions, such as hepatic ascites, where hypokalaemia is particularly dangerous. In fact, hyperkalaemia may occur when it is used alone. It sometimes produces nausea, vomiting and diarrhoea.

(f) *Amiloride*. This drug resembles triameterene in its structure, pharmacology, therapeutic indications and adverse effects. When given with thiazide diuretics it potentiates sodium excretion and reduces potassium loss. Excessive sodium and water loss may lead to an increase in blood urea and vascular collapse. Dangerous hyperkalaemia can occur.

(g) *Carbonic anhydrase inhibitors*. In the proximal and distal tubules sodium ions are exchanged for hydrogen ions generated from H_2O and CO_2 under the influence of the enzyme carbonic anhydrase. Inhibition of this enzyme with drugs such as acetazolamide reduces the availability of hydrogen ions and so leads to an increase in excretion of sodium together with bicarbonate with the production of an alkaline urine. The increase in bicarbonate excretion leads to a metabolic acidosis which in turn reduces the effectiveness of the drug. The action of acetazolamide may disappear therefore, after only 48 hours of treatment. For this reason it has been largely superseded by the thiazides and other diuretics. Toxic effects include drowsiness, mental confusion and paraesthesiae of the extremities.

Osmotic diuretics

Active sodium reabsorption in the proximal tubule is accompanied by absorption of isosmotic amounts of water. The administration of an osmotic diuretic and its presence in the lumen of the renal tubule opposes this reabsorption of water and, indirectly, reduces sodium reabsorption. Apart from this action, some of the osmotic diuretics such as mannitol, also improve renal perfusion.

Mannitol, a non-metabolized sugar alcohol, is the most important of this group of agents. It is administered intravenously in concentrations of 5 to 20 per cent and is freely filtered at the glomerulus. It is not reabsorbed by the tubules, and so has been used to measure the glomerular filtration rate. The infusion must be carefully monitored as it may lead to increased circulating volume and central venous pressure, cardiac failure, plasma hyperosmolality and hyponatraemia. Indications for treatment with mannitol are:

(a) Oedema refractory to other diuretics given alone or in combination. In such cases it may initiate a diuresis which is then maintained by other agents.

(b) Drug poisoning where a forced diuresis increases the rate of elimimation.

(c) To improve renal blood flow in conditions where renal failure might occur, such as shock and in cardiovascular surgery.

Potassium supplements

Although potassium loss may lead to a severe degree of hypokalaemia with its associated muscle weakness, mental disturbances, cardiac effects, and, in patients with hepatic ascites, risk of encephalopathy, the true risk of this happening as a result of diuretic treatment is controversial. There is no doubt about its importance in patients receiving digitalis for heart disease, in whom hypokalaemia increases the risk of digitalis intoxication. It is also more likely to occur in the elderly, particularly those with poor dietary habits. In general, however, the risks to a patient from hyperkalaemia are greater than those from hypokalaemia, except in patients receiving digitalis, and the routine use of potassium supplements wherever a thiazide-type or loop diuretic is being used is clinically unwise. Potassium loss associated with use of these diuretics may be reduced by combined treatment with a potassium sparing diuretic such as spironolactone, triamterene or amiloride. However, these drugs carry the hazard of hyperkalaemia particularly when potassium supplements are also given.

When treatment with potassium supplements is indicated, potassium chloride is the compound of choice since chloride is required to correct the alkalosis that accompanies the hypokalaemia. In solution potassium chloride is poorly tolerated because of its nauseous effects, and other formulations have therefore been introduced which are better tolerated. Slow-release preparations, in which potassium chloride diffuses out of a wax matrix as it passes through the small intestine, appear to be relatively safe compared with earlier enteric-coated formulations which were associated with hazards of small bowel necrosis, ulceration, perforation and stricture. An effervescent preparation containing betaine hydrochloride and potassium bicarbonate is available and appears to be well tolerated and effective.

The normal diet contains about 80–100 mEq daily of potassium.

Slow release preparations such as Slow-K contain about 8 mEq potassium, so that 10 daily would be required to provide this intake, although such doses are seldom used. Clinical hypokalaemia probably requires doses in excess of 60–80 mEq daily, and it may then be more convenient to use 10% potassium chloride elixir because of its rapid absorption from the stomach. Daily oral doses in excess of 100 mEq should only be administered with great caution because of the cardiac risks of hyperkalaemia.

Intravenous administration of potassium chloride should only be carried out slowly under constant supervision for evidence of cardiac dysrhythmias. It should not exceed a rate of 20 mmol per hour or a concentration of 50 mmol per litre.

11

Drugs and the respiratory system

Respiratory centre

Stimulation. There is a variety of compounds which stimulate the respiratory and cardiovascular centres in the midbrain and hypothalamus. They were widely used to stimulate respiration in patients with respiratory depression due to drugs or disease, but with the development of mechanical devices for artificial ventilation they are now seldom employed. Their therapeutic ratio is generally low, and overdosage induces convulsions and delirium. Among the more important of these compounds are pentylenetetrazol, bemegride, nikethamide, doxapram and picrotoxin.

Depression. A wide range of central nervous depressant drugs produce respiratory depression when administered in excess of their therapeutic doses, including barbiturates, alcohol and the narcotic analgesic drugs.

Drugs and the bronchus

The pharmacology of bronchial smooth muscle is summarized in Table 12.

Table 12 Pharmacology of bronchial muscle

Neurogenic	Constriction	Dilatation
Parasympathetic	+	
Sympathetic		+
Autonomic receptor		
Cholinergic	+	
Adrenergic α	+	
β_2		+
Histamine	+	
5-Hydroxytryptamine	+	
Others		
Kinins	+	
SRS-A	+	
Prostaglandins	+	+

Bronchospastic drugs

Bronchoconstriction may be produced by acetylcholine, muscarine, histamine, 5-hydroxytryptamine, bradykinin and slow-reacting substance (SRS) all of which produce spasm of bronchial smooth muscle. There is also evidence that some prostaglandins may possess bronchoconstrictor and some bronchodilator properties. The role of one or more of these pharmacological agents in bronchial asthma is still uncertain.

β-Adrenoceptor blocking drugs may produce bronchoconstriction by preventing sympathetically mediated bronchodilator tone (p. 51).

Bronchodilators

(a) *Sympathomimetic amines.* Sympathetic stimulation produces bronchodilatation through β-receptor activity, and therefore β-receptor agonists such as isoprenaline and orciprenaline are potent bronchodilators compared with noradrenaline which primarily activates α-adrenergic receptors. Adrenaline, which has marked affinity for both α- and β-receptors, is also a potent bronchodilator drug. These drugs stimulate β-receptors generally and therefore increase the rate and force of cardiac contraction in doses which dilate the bronchi.

Selective β_2-receptor agonists such as isoetharine, salbutamol, rimiterol and terbutaline dilate the bronchi and reduce the bronchoconstrictor effects of histamine and acetylcholine in doses which do not produce any cardiac effects. Higher doses, however, do produce cardiac stimulation and tremor, and these drugs should therefore be used with caution in patients with underlying heart disease. Although some may be administered orally and parenterally, the most convenient route is by inhalation from fixed and fewer adverse effects occur with this route of administration. The bronchodilator action appears rapidly within minutes of inhalation and may persist for some hours.

(b) *Xanthines.* These drugs act by inhibiting phosphodiesterase and hence have actions which resemble sympathetic stimulation, but are not blocked by adrenergic neurone or receptor blocking drugs. Aminophylline, which is a combination of theophylline and ethylenediamine, has useful bronchodilator properties in conditions such as bronchial asthma and pulmonary oedema where bronchoconstriction is present. It can be given intravenously in status asthmaticus, but slow administration is necessary because of the danger of cardiac dysrhythmias and fits. By suppository it is erratically absorbed. Theophylline and aminophylline are now available is slow release oral preparations which produce sustained therapeutic plasma levels for up to 10–12 hours and need only to be administered every 12 hours. They should replace older preparations such as choline theophyllinate which produce adequate plasma levels for only a few hours and have a higher incidence of gastric irritation.

(c) *Anticholinergic drugs.* Drugs which block the muscarinic actions of acetylcholine, such as atropine, have bronchodilator properties, and the increase in airway resistance produced in asthmatic and bronchitic patients by aerosols of histamine or carbon dust is abolished by the administration of atropine methonitrate. It is, therefore, included in some aerosol preparations with sympathomimetic amines. Although its bronchodilator action may be an advantage, it also reduces the volume of secretions in the bronchial tree, resulting in decreased fluidity and increased viscosity. The secretions may then be more difficult to expectorate, leading to obstructed airflow and pulmonary infection. These effects may more than outweigh any advantage gained by using atropine in bronchial asthma.

Deptropine and ipratropium are recently introduced anticholinergic drugs they are probably effective than the β_2-receptor agonists such as salbutamol in asthma, but appear to be as effective in patients with chronic bronchitis who have reversible airway obstruction. Effects on sputum viscosity appear to be unimportant.

Disodium cromoglycate

This drug is not a bronchodilator, nor does it antagonize mediators of tissue reaction such as histamine or slow-reacting substance. Its main action is prophylactic, reducing the incidence and severity of allergic asthmatic attacks, and the dosage of corticosteroids and bronchodilator drugs required by asthmatic patients. Its value in the treatment of acute attacks is not well established. The mechanism of its action is uncertain, but it may involve inhibition of release of histamine and slow-reacting substance from the mast cells by stabilisation of the mast cell membrane, so preventing exocytosis (p. 36).

Disodium cromoglycate is a powder, poorly absorbed from the gut. It is, therefore, administered by inhalation from a special dispenser, a spinhaler, in which a propeller activated by suction creates a cloud of powder from the punctured capsule in which it is contained. Isoprenaline is included in some preparations to protect against bronchospasm caused by inhalation of a dry powder. It may also be of value in other conditions with an allergic basis, such as hay fever, allergic conjunctivitis, aphthous ulceration and lactose intolerance.

Ketotifen

Ketotifen combines antihistamine with anti-allergic properties similar to those of disodium cromoglycate, but has the advantage that it is active after oral ingestion. Its role in management of asthma and other allergic conditions is being assessed. Its most common adverse effect is sedation which can occur even at therapeutic doses.

Bronchial asthma

Bronchial asthma has two principal components, increased tone of the smooth muscle within the bronchial walls, and increased secretion by mucosal glands. These two factors may be produced experimentally by a variety of substances such as histamine, slow-reacting substance (SRS-A) and 5-hydroxytryptamine, some of which may be responsible in part for allergic forms of the condition. Parasympathetic activity, mediated by release of acetylcholine, also produces increased tone and secretion, and may be responsible for asthmatic attacks triggered off by psychogenic stimuli.

Prophylaxis. The incidence and severity of attacks may be reduced by regular administration of (a) disodium cromoglycate which interferes with the allergic response, (b) bronchodilator drugs such as the sympathomimetic amines ephedrine given orally, orciprenaline given orally or by aerosol, and salbutamol given orally or by aerosol. Xanthines such as theophylline and its derivatives may be given orally. Adjusting the dose to produce a serum level of 40 to 100 μmol/l (9 to 18 μg/ml) has been shown to give an optimum bronchodilator effect. (c) corticosteroids. Oral treatment with prednisolone or other corticosteroids is often effective, but is associated with the risk of adrenal suppression with its ensuing complications (p. 204). Beclomethasone and betamethasone are administered by aerosol and have been shown to have prophylactic value, without producing significant adrenal suppression in usual therapeutic doses. They may, however, be associated with fungal infections of the trachea and bronchi.

Treatment of acute attack. While some authorities still advocate the use of subcutaneous adrenaline in the acute asthmatic attack, it is now becoming accepted practice to begin treatment in hospital with inhaled salbutamol administered through a ventilator such as the Bird model. Aminophylline may be given very slowly over 10 to 15 minutes by intravenous injection or by infusion, with continuous monitoring of the heart rate. Intravenous hydrocortisone in high doses is also given followed by oral prednisolone, again in high dosage. Oxygen is given as required, in a concentration not exceeding 35 per cent. A marked respiratory acidosis is often found in severe asthmatic attacks, and this may contribute to resistance to the bronchodilator action of drugs such as adrenaline and salbutamol. It is important, therefore, to correct any acid-base disturbance which occurs. If the patient does not respond satisfactorily to these measures, intubation, or even tracheostomy, with assisted or controlled ventilation should be considered.

Dangers of excessive aerosal usage. Following reports of an increase in the number of children dying from asthma in Great Britain between 1960 and 1965, it was suggested that this might be associated with excessive use of sympathomimetic agents in the form of metered or pressurized aerosols of isoprenaline, orciprenaline or adrenaline. A comprehensive analysis has demonstrated a marked correlation between sales and prescriptions of these formulations over the years 1960 to 1967 and deaths from asthma, and has also shown that as the sale of pressurized aerosols began to fall from 1966, so the mortality curve has shown a sharp decline. Although the sympathomimetic amines might be considered to be the most likely agents responsible for the toxicity of these preparations in view of their known cardiotoxic effects, the possibility must be considered that the fluorinated methane and ethane derivatives which are commonly used as aerosol propellants may play a part. There have been reports of deaths in young people who inhaled these fluorocarbons for their central stimulant effects, and it has been suggested that these substances can sensitize the myocardium to circulating catecholamines during hypoxia and produce a cardiac dysrthythmia. Estimations of these propellants, however, from chronic overusers of such bronchodilator aerosols have shown that the blood levels reached are probably not high enough to produce such myocardial sensitization. It seems probable that many of the deaths occurring in the nineteen-sixties, and indeed that still occur, resulted from complacency on the part of patients, relatives and doctors because of an unwarrented confidence in the new sympathominetic drugs, and from inadequate management, particularly in the use of steroids.

Expectorants
Expectorants are used in inflammatory conditions of the respiratory tract and are claimed to increase the volume of bronchial secretion, and render it less tenacious. In general they are emetic compounds

administered in subemetic doses, emesis being preceded by increased activity of secretory glands. The most commonly used are standard formulations of sodium chloride, ipecacuanha, ammonium chloride, potassium iodide, and squill. They are relatively harmless in standard doses, although chronic ingestion of potassium iodide by patients with asthma and bronchitis may lead to thyroid suppression, and if taken by women during pregnancy may produce congenital goitre and hypothyroidism in the newborn. Bromhexine is a synthetic drug which has been shown to increase sputum volume and decrease its viscosity.

Cough suppressants

Cough suppressants, or antitussive agents, are used in the symptomatic treatment of cough. They are of two types:

(a) Drugs which are used primarily to relieve pain, but which also depress respiration and suppress the cough reflex. Among the more important of these is the opium alkaloid, codeine, and the synthetic compounds pholcodine and dextromethorphan.

(b) Drugs which specifically raise the threshold of the cough centre in the brain or which act peripherally to reduce the afferent flow of impulses which stimulate the cough centre. Noscapine, also derived from opium, resembles papaverine in its action on smooth muscle, and has cough suppressant properties while lacking the narcotic effect of morphine and its related compounds. Several of the drugs in this group such as benzonatate, carbetapentane and dimethoxanate have local anaesthetic, atropine-like or antispasmodic properties which probably contribute to their therapeutic effect.

12

Drugs on the Gastrointestinal tract

The stomach and intestines have a dual autonomic innervation. The parasympathetic division is responsible for secretion of digestive enzymes, peristalsis and relaxation of sphincters, whereas the sympathetic system produces effects opposite to these. Thus cholinomimetic drugs and anticholinesterases will cause colic and promote defaecation, while anticholinergic drugs relax the bowel and cause constipation. Drugs which block autonomic ganglia reduce both the sympathetic and parasympathetic drive, but constipation ensues as parasympathetic activity is normally predominant. Drugs which selectively block sympathetic nerve terminals, e.g. bethanidine, often cause diarrhoea. Sympathomimetic drugs act on the bowel mainly through α-receptors, but this has little practical significance.

Gastrointestinal secretions can be reduced in volume by anticholinergic drugs, but the treatment of peptic ulcer with these compounds is limited. A more promising approach is the possible use of an antihistamine which specifically blocks gastric H_2 receptors.

DRUGS IN PEPTIC ULCER

Antacids

Antacids are weak bases which react with hydrochloric acid in the stomach to form a salt. This salt should preferably be non-absorbable, for if it is absorbed, systemic alkalosis can result. This is the major drawback with sodium bicarbonate.

The object of treatment is to produce a prolonged increase in the pH of the stomach, but in practice this is seldom achieved because large quantities (1500 ml) of gastric juice are produced daily, and up to 60 g of sodium bicarbonate per day would be required to usefully reduce its acidity (a pH above 4·0). In addition, antacids often provoke gastric acid production, leading to an 'acid rebound'. This is particularly marked with calcium salts. All available antacids have too short a duration of action to reduce the acidity of the stomach for long after a single dose. This can be overcome either by an intragastric drip of milk or milk-alkali mixture, or by the use of Nulacin or Prodexin tablets, which are designed to be sucked, and slowly release the antacids which they contain.

Antacids are useful for reducing the pain of uncomplicated peptic ulceration or oesophagitis but they promote healing of ulcers only when given in doses in excess of 1000 μmol daily, quantities which frequently produce diarrhoea. They help little in other forms of indigestion, although the belching promoted by carbon dioxide released from sodium bicarbonate gives relief to some patients. Belching can also be promoted by polymethylsiloxane, an antifoaming agent.

Sodium bicarbonate. This is rapidly effective in relieving ulcer pain, and is a component of many popular proprietary antacid mixtures. Systemic alkalosis occurs when large doses are taken daily. This leads to excretion of a persistently alkaline urine, which can disturb excretion of other drugs and of calcium. If large quantities of milk or calcium-containing antacid are taken simultaneously, hypercalcaemia and renal calcinosis can occur ('milk-alkali' syndrome). The use of sodium bicarbonate in patients with hypertension, congestive cardiac failure or renal disease is unwise, for the sodium load can be substantial.

Calcium carbonate. This is an effective antacid and produces a more prolonged reduction in gastric acidity than sodium bicarbonate. Calcium soaps are formed in the intestine by combination with fatty acids. Frequent use can cause constipation.

Magnesium hydroxide. Interaction with gastric acid produces magnesium chloride, which is poorly absorbed but soluble. It acts as an osmotic purgative, as does magnesium sulphate. This is the reason why magnesium antacids are often mixed with constipating calcium or aluminium antacids. The action of magnesium hydroxide is slower and more prolonged than that of sodium bicarbonate.

Magnesium trisilicate. Magnesium chloride and hydrated silicic acid are formed when this substance reacts with gastric acid. The silicic acid is gelatinous in consistency and has good adsorbent properties, which enhance the antacid effect. Its onset of action, however, is slow.

Aluminium hydroxide. This has both antacid and adsorbent properties. Aluminium ions cause constipation by an inhibitory action on intestinal smooth muscle. They also inhibit pepsin, although this does not produce any appreciable change in protein digestion. Phosphate ions are bound as insoluble salts, and this can produce hypophosphataemia. Aluminium compounds are sometimes used for this purpose in hyperphosphataemia accompanying renal failure. Tetracycline absorption can be impaired by chelation.

In practice, one of the most satisfactory preparations combining high neutralizing capacity, a rapid but long-lasting effect, absence of rebound hypersecretion, non-absorbability, palatability and safety is a liquid mixture of equal parts of magnesium trisilicate and aluminium hydroxide.

Anticholinergic drugs

Anticholinergic drugs can reduce the volume of gastric acid secreted, but have little or no effect on the pH of the empty stomach. After a meal, however, the acidity of the stomach can be decreased by anticholinergics, but the effect is small, for acid production at this time is largely the result of food-stimulated gastrin secretion. In some ulcer patients symptoms may be caused partly by disturbances of gastric motility and muscle spasm, and anticholinergics may help to overcome this.

Unwanted effects are usual in the dosage required to reduce gastric motility, and are the result of peripheral anticholinergic effects. They should not be used in patients with reflux oesophagitis, pyloric stenosis, glaucoma or prostatic hypertrophy.

There is probably little difference between the various anticholinergic drugs, although hyoscine butylbromide, propantheline and poldine have been the most popular for use in peptic ulcer. H_2-receptor blocking drugs have now largely supplanted their use. Dicyclomine is used for infantile pyloric stenosis and evening colic.

H_2-receptor blocking drugs

Histamine is a powerful stimulant of gastric acid secretion but this effect is not blocked by the traditional antihistamines, which act on H_1-receptors. This differential effect has been utilized in the augmented histamine test, in which the ability of the gastric mucosa to secrete acid is tested by administration of a large dose of histamine plus the antihistamine, mepyramine maleate. It has been suggested that histamine might act as a final common pathway in the secretion of gastric acid, whether it is provoked by gastrin, the synthetic analogue pentagastrin, or by vagus nerve stimulation (e.g. sight or smell of food). This theory is supported by the observation that metiamide and cimetidine, H_2-receptor blocking drugs, powerfully suppress the acid secretion produced by all these stimuli. Acid secretion in ulcer patients is likewise reduced, leading not only to symptomatic relief but also to healing of the ulcer.

Clinical trials have shown that cimetidine promotes the healing of both gastric and duodenal ulcers, and controls peptic ulceration in the Zollinger-Ellison syndrome. Oesophagitis is also improved. A four to six week treatment period is followed by maintenance therapy in a lower dose. Withdrawal of treatment is often followed by a relapse, but there is no evidence of rebound hypersecretion. Cimetidine has no functional effect on the course of the disease.

Liquorice derivatives

Extraction of liquorice root yields glycyrrhizinic acid and a variety of residues. These derivatives form the basis of two proprietary preparations. Carbenoxolone sodium is a derivative of glycyrrhizinic acid, and 'Caved-S' contains liquorice residues (deglycyrrhizinized liquorice) as well as several antacids. Both these substances promote healing of gastric ulcers, and when given in positioned-release capsules which burst on passing through the pylorus, healing of duodenal ulcers also occurs. Their therapeutic effect may be due to a number of factors, including an increase in the life span of gastric epithelial cells, an increase in mucus production and a change in its composition, a decrease in hydrogen-ion back-diffusion and an inhibition of peptic activity.

The main difference between these two derivatives lies in their systemic effects. Carbenoxolone has anti-inflammatory properties, partly by stimulation of adrenocortical steroid production. Aldosterone-like effects cause potassium loss, and retention of sodium and chloride. Hypokalaemia can cause lassitude and weakness, and sodium retention can precipitate oedema and heart failure. The drug should therefore not be used in the old and those with heart or renal disease. A sodium-depleting, potassium-retaining diuretic will reverse these effects, but spironolactone also antagonizes the ulcer-healing action. A thiazide diuretic can aggravate hypokalaemia. Plasma potassium should be measured frequently, and potassium supplements given if necessary. Maintenance treatment is impracticable because of the risks of electrolyte imbalance.

Deglycyrrhizinized liquorice does not have these effects, although diarrhoea occasionally occurs.

Chelated bismuth

Chelated bismuth salts promote healing of gastric and duodenal ulcer ulcers, possibly by coating the crater. No important adverse effects have been reported.

Drugs affecting gastric emptying

Anticholinergic drugs such as propantheline delay gastric emptying by reducing parasympathetic tone. The absorption of other drugs given concurrently, e.g. paracetamol, can be delayed by this effect. Tricyclic antidepressants, phenothiazines, antihistamines and anti-Parkinsonian drugs are likely to have similar effects as they often have marked anticholinergic actions. On the other hand, metoclopramide promotes gastric emptying and can speed up drug absorption. This effect is taken advantage of during barium meal estimations.

Enzymes and bile salts

Pancreatin. This is an extract of hog pancreas, and contains amylase, trypsin and lipase. It is used in patients who have steatorrhoea from pancreatic disease, but it is of little value unless protected from gastric acid either by using a preparation with an enteric coating or by giving large doses of antacids at the same time.

Bile salts. Dehydrocholic acid increases the volume of bile produced by the liver, but not its content of bile salts. It is of limited value and may aggravate pruritus in biliary stasis.

Cholestyramine. This is an anion-exchange resin which removes bile anions in exchange for chloride ions, and can be of value in reducing the pruritus which accompanies biliary cirrhosis and obstructive jaundice. It also lowers the serum cholesterol (bile salts are formed from cholesterol) but this is usually only temporary.

Chenodeoxycholic acid. Cholesterol gall stones occur when bile contains an excess of cholesterol relative to its bile salt and phospholipid content. Chenodeoxycholic acid alters this ratio in favour of bile salts and phospholipids. It dissolves established gall-stones and prevents their recurrence. It also reduces plasma triglyceride levels. Chenodeoxycholic acid is metabolised in the liver to lithocholic acid, which is hepatotoxic.

Cation-exchange resins

These compounds comprise an insoluble polystyrene matrix with an attached, permanently bound anion. The anion attracts cations, but the latter are free to exchange with other cations in the vicinity. Thus a resin given in the H^+ or NH_4^+ form (Katonium) will remove sodium ions on its passage through the gut. This substance was much used in treating resistant oedema, but it has been displaced by potent thiazide diuretics.

In acute renal failure potassium retention occurs, but this can be corrected by an oral Na^+ resin (Resonium A). However, continuous use of this can lead to hypernatraemia, with hypertension and oedema. Calcium Resonium overcomes this problem, but even though calcium ions are poorly absorbed hypercalcaemia can occur. An aluminium resin may be preferable.

Purgatives

The terms 'purgative', 'laxative', 'aperient' and 'cathartic' should be regarded as synonymous, as attempts at a classification using these terms lead to confusion. 'Purgatives' can be divided into three types according to their mode of action, (a) bulk purgatives, (b) lubricant purgatives, and (c) irritant purgatives.

Bulk purgatives

These act by increasing the bulk of the intestinal contents, promoting normal peristalsis and defaecation. Three types are available.

(a) Osmotic purgatives, which include salts having a non-absorbable ion, such as magnesium in magnesium sulphate (Epsom salts) or sulphate in sodium sulphate (Glauber's salts) and the polysaccharide, lactulose. They retain water by osmosis, providing liquid bulk.

(b) Hydrophilic colloids, such as methylcellulose, agar or psyllium, which are indigestible plant residues which absorb water, swell, and increase faecal bulk.

(c) Vegetable fibres, such as bran, which are also indigestible and provide bulk, but are not colloidal. Large doses have produced intestinal obstruction.

Lubricant purgatives

Liquid paraffin is the most important example. It lubricates faecal material in the colon and rectum, and can be useful when straining is undesirable or when defaecation is painful, as in anal fissure or following haemorrhoidectomy, although it can delay healing after anal surgery. It reduces absorption of the fat-soluble vitamins A and D, and can cause paraffinomas in mesenteric lymph nodes with chronic use. It may leak from the anal sphincter. There is a danger of aspiration pneumonia in the elderly.

Dioctyl sodium sulphosuccinate is a newer substance which lowers surface tension, allowing water to penetrate and soften the faecal matter. Its effect is limited.

Glycerine suppositories and soft soap enemata have long been used as local lubricants.

Irritant purgatives

The drugs included in this group act in a variety of ways, for which the descriptive term 'irritant' is an oversimplification. Anthracene derivatives, including senna and cascara, are hydrolyzed to trihyd-roxymethyl anthraquinone (emodin) which stimulates Auerbach's plexus in the bowel wall. They may produce a reddish-brown dis-colouration of the urine, and are excreted in the milk of lactating mothers. Castor oil is hydrolyzed also, producing ricinoleic acid, which is irritant to the small bowel. Bisacodyl probably acts by stimulating sensory nerve endings in the mucosa of the large bowel. It can be taken orally or given as a suppository. Phenolphthalein, and a more potent chemically-related compound, oxyphenisatin, stimulate the colonic smooth muscle directly. They are absorbed and reexcreted in bile, and this 'entero-hepatic' circulation prolongs their action. Phenolphthalein sensitivity occasionally occurs, lead-ing to a blotchy rash. A variety of 'drastic' purgatives, such as cro-ton oil and jalap, are extremely irritant and are no longer used.

Indications and adverse effects
Fortunately the fashion for regular use of purgatives is on the decline. There is no justification for the use of these drugs in the normal person. Variation in the frequency of defaecation and in the consistency of the faeces is a normal phenomenon, and not an indi-cation for purgation. Usually the administration of a purgative will exaggerate this variation, for complete emptying of the large bowel is usually followed by a period of two or three days without defae-cation. The person who is overconcerned about his bowel habit will see this period as a justification for his regular use of a purgative.

Purgation is indicated in the following situations:

(a) In bowel disease accompanied by chronic constipation e.g. megacolon without aganglionosis.

(b) In the treatment of helmintic infections of the bowel.

(c) Before surgery on the large bowel and rectum. Senna and cascara, which act on the large bowel, are suitable for this.

(d) Before sigmoidoscopy or radiology of the bowel, although an enema may be more effective.

(e) In local disease of the anus or rectum, such as haemorrhoids or anal fissure. Liquid paraffin is most used in this situation.

(f) Following ingestion of poisons.

(g) In constipation produced by drugs, such as opiates and seda-tives.

(h) In hepatic encephalopathy.

Most of the irritant purgatives are slow to act, and are given usually last thing at night. Where rapid purgation is required, e.g. after ingestion of poisons, osmotic purgatives are best.

Purgation can produce many adverse effects. Colicky abdominal pain is frequent, and diarrhoea can follow, leading to dehydration and electrolyte imbalance. Chronic purgation can cause diarrhoea, weight loss, hypokalaemia and muscle weakness. Damage to the myenteric plexus of the large bowel can occur. Acute and chronic active hepatitis have been described with purgatives containing oxyphenisatin. Purgatives should never be given to a patient with undiagnosed abdominal pain, for they can precipitate dangerous complications, e.g. burst appendix.

Antidiarrhoeal drugs

Symptomatic treatment for diarrhoea can be given by administering either an adsorbent substance, which adsorbs irritants, or a drug which alters the tone and motility of the bowel. The cause of the diarrhoea should be considered, and specific therapy given at the same time, if indicated. In acute diarrhoea, antibiotics should be administered only if justified on bacteriological grounds. A severe bacterial infection is best treated with systemic antibiotics (e.g. ampicillin) rather than locally-acting non-absorbed compounds (e.g. neomycin).

Charcoal, chalk and kaolin are the most used adsorbents, although pectin is also of value. Kaolin and morphine mixture remains the most popular antidiarrhoeal preparation.

Opiates increase smooth muscle tone in the bowel, and reduce its motility. This property makes them valuable anti-diarrhoeal drugs. Morphine and codeine phosphate are the most used for this purpose, as most of the synthetic or semisynthetic derivatives have less effect on the bowel. One exception is diphenoxylate, a derivative of pethidine, which is contained in a popular proprietary preparation (Lomotil). Loperamide is related to diphenoxylate, but inhibits colonic activity partly by reducing acetylcholine release from parasympathetic terminals in the bowel wall. The dose of morphine required to counteract diarrhoea is small, and systemic effects are rare. Codeine phosphate, however, sometimes produces dizziness and nausea.

Anticholinergic drugs are often included in antidiarrhoeal preparations, although their use is probably irrational, as diarrhoea often results not from excessive peristaltic activity, but from lack of segmental contractions which delay the passage of the bowel contents. A low dose of atropine is included in some preparations (e.g. Lomotil) in order to lessen abuse.

13

Drugs on appetite and weight

OBESITY

Medical treatment of obesity depends on the principle that weight loss can only occur when calorie intake falls below calorie expenditure. There is no substitute for this principle, and drugs which are prescribed to produce weight loss or assist dietary management must depend on influencing calorie intake or expenditure.

Increased calorie expenditure

Thyroid hormones in the form of thyroid extract or L-thyroxine are still used by many doctors to increase metabolic rate and produce weight loss. This is undesirable, however, as the doses of these drugs required to produce weight loss may also produce clinical signs of thyroid overactivity and lead to the development of angina pectoris in patients with ischaemic heart disease.

There is evidence that some anorectic drugs such as fenfluramine, mazindol and the biguanides may in addition have metabolic effects increasing calorie expenditure. The relative importance of appetite-suppressing and metabolic actions in producing their therapeutic effects, however, is uncertain.

Reduction of food intake

There have been sporadic attempts to reduce the absorption of food from the intestine by short-circuiting operations which produce a malabsorption state. These are not satisfactory, however, as they may lead to chronic malnutrition and vitamin deficiencies which are not acceptable alternatives to obesity.

(a) Bulk agents

If hunger results from gastric emptiness, then it is reasonable to suppose that ingestion of inert substances which are not absorbed from the gut would relieve hunger without providing calories for weight increase. The most commonly used substance is methylcellulose which is available as tablets or in various food substitutes. Although free from adverse side-effects, its therapeutic value has not been proven satisfactory.

(b) Anorectic drugs

Appetite suppression result from a sensation of satiety which, in turn, depends on the activity of the 'satiety' centre in the ventromedial hypothalamus. This centre can be suppressed by a variety of drugs.

1. Sympathomimetic amines. Indirectly acting amines such as amphetamine and its derivatives dexamphetamine, phenmetrazine, diethylpropion, chlorphentermine and phentermine, assist patients to adhere to a dietary regime and to lose weight. They are most effective if taken 1– 1½ hours before a meal and controlled studies using linear analogue rating scales have demonstrated a significant reduction in appetite by these drugs. Their most important adverse effect is central stimulation, with restlessness, anxiety, insomnia, tolerance and habituation. They are most marked with amphetamine, dexamphetamine and phenmetrazine. This has resulted in considerable abuse of these compounds with legislation restricting their availability in some countries. There is now general agreement that they should not be prescribed in conditions for which there is alternative treatment without such adverse effects. It was believed that appetite suppression might be inevitably linked with central stimulation. This is now known not to be so, as a trifluoromethyl derivative of amphetamine, fenfluramine, has anorectic and weight-reducing properties without producing central stimulation. In fact, it may produce sedation in therapeutic doses, particularly in anxious patients. It is probable that the central actions of fenfluramine are mediated through 5HT mechanisms rather than through noradrenergic or dopaminergic mechanisms as with the amphetamines. Metabolic studies in animals and man suggest that fenfluramine may have fat mobilizing effects and increase glucose uptake in skeletal muscle, in addition to its anorectic action. Mazindol is an indole derivative which blocks neuronal reuptake of dopamine and noradrenaline and has anorectic activity.

2. Biguanides. These drugs, of which metformin and phenformin are the principal members in current use, are alternatives to the sulphonylurea compounds in the oral treatment of diabetes. They frequently produce anorexia both in diabetic and nondiabetic patients and for this reason may be the drugs of choice in the overweight maturity-onset diabetic patient who is unable to adhere to a diet or in whom diet alone has failed to produce satisfactory weight loss. It is probable that other metabolic effects contribute to their weight reducing properties.

STIMULATION OF APPETITE

It is sometimes desirable in clinical practice to increase appetite and body weight. Cyproheptadine is an antihistamine and 5HT antagonist which was noticed to increase appetite and weight during an evaluation of its effect on childhood asthma. Its mode of action is obscure and its metabolic effects and the nature of the weight gain are poorly understood.

14

Antidiabetic drugs

Insulin is released from the β-cells of the islets of the pancreas in response to hyperglycaemia. It seems likely that cyclic AMP is the mediator of this effect in the pancreatic cells, and this would account for the influence of other hormones on insulin release.

Insulin is a polypeptide, made up of two chains of amino acids linked by two disulphide bridges. The sequence of amino acids has been elucidated, and this has lead to its synthesis, but for medical use insulin is still extracted from pork or beef pancreas. The insulins from these two species are identical except for one terminal amino acid, but this difference is important when antibody production occurs to one of the two, for then the other may be able to be substituted without cross-immunity.

Insulin exerts its effects by stimulating intracellular synthesis of glycogen, thus facilitating transport of glucose across the cell membrane. It also increases the production of cell proteins and promotes fat storage in adipose tissue. The insulin-stimulated transport of glucose is accompanied by a movement of potassium ions into the cell, and this has been used to reduce the plasma potassium level in hyperkalaemia. Hypokalaemia is rapidly produced by insulin treatment of diabetic coma, and this makes it imperative that repeated estimations of the plasma potassium level are made during the early stages of treatment. Intravenous potassium chloride is usually needed to maintain the plasma level.

Although the physiological secretion of insulin amounts to less than 50 units/day, often much larger doses than this have to be administered to a diabetic patient because antibodies are formed within the first few weeks of treatment, particularly with beef insulin, resulting in the formation of antigen-antibody complexes.

Insulin has to be given by injection, because, being a polypeptide, it is digested by proteolytic enzymes in the gut.

Choice of insulins
When pure, insulin has a very low antigenicity. The immunogenic

properties of standard insulins are mainly caused by small amounts of protein impurities, particularly pro-insulin, derived from the pancreas. In order to overcome this problem, two types of purified insulin have been developed: *pro-insulin freed*, and *highly purified* (sometimes known as *monocomponent* or *rarely-immunogenic*). Unfortunately, the introduction of these new preparations has led to confusion as similar names are used for insulins of different grades of purity. Trade names have therefore been used in Table 13, in order to lessen confusion.

Table 13   Insulins

Preparation	Composition	Duration of action (hr)	Number of doses per day
(a) Standard (beef)			
Soluble	Acidic solution of insulin	8	Two or more
Neutral	Neutral solution of insulin	8	Two or more
Zinc suspension semilente[a]	Amorphous suspension + zinc	16	Two
Zinc suspension lente	3 parts semilente + 7 parts ultralente	30	One or two
Zinc suspension ultralente	Crystalline suspension + zinc	36	One or two
Protamine zinc	Insulin-protamine complex in suspension + zinc	48	One
Globin zinc	Insulin solution with globin + zinc		
Isophane (NPH)	Insulin-protamine complex + zinc		Now little used
(b) Pro-insulin freed			
Rapitard[b]	Soluble pork insulin + long-acting beef insulin	30	One or two
Lentard[b]	Equivalent to zinc suspension lente (beef + pork)	30	One or two
Ultratard[b]	Equivalent to zinc suspension ultralente (beef)	36	One or two
(c) Highly purified (pork)			
Actrapid MC[b]	Equivalent to soluble	7	Two or more
Leo Neutral[b]	Equivalent to neutral	8	Two or more
Semitard MC[b]	Equivalent to zinc suspension semilente	15	Two or more
Monotard MC[b]	Equivalent to zinc suspension lente	20	One or two
Leo Retard[b]	Equivalent to isophane (NPH)	24	One or two

[a] Zinc suspension semilente made by Novo is pro-insulin freed pork insulin.
[b] Trade names have been used to avoid confusion.

Standard insulins are usually slightly longer-acting than their purified equivalents because they are derived from beef insulin, which is more immunogenic than pork insulin, and the resulting antigen-antibody complexes only gradually release active insulin. Pro-insulin freed preparations are less immunogenic than standard insulins, but are more so than highly purified preparations, which are derived from pork insulin and which are claimed to evoke little or no antibody formation. As a result, these latter preparations are shorter acting.

The dose requirements of highly purified insulins are lower than for standard insulins, and allowance needs to be made for this if a patient is changed from the latter to the former. Highly purified insulins provoke fewer allergic reactions, do not cause fat necrosis at injection sites, and avoid the formation of IgG insulin antibodies during pregnancy which can cross the placenta and reach the foetus.

Insulin preparations can be sub-divided according to their duration of action:

(a) *Short-acting*. Soluble insulins act within 30 minutes after subcutaneous injection, but can be given intravenously to produce a rapid effect in an emergency. Stabilization on soluble insulin alone requires frequent injections, and therefore it is more usual to combine it with a longer-acting preparation, e.g lente insulin.

(b) *Medium-acting*. Semilente preparations have a slower onset of action than soluble insulin but their duration of action extends to 15 to 16 hours.

(c) *Long-acting*. Ultralente insulins are very slow in onset of action (6 to 8 hours). Lente preparations begin their effects earlier (2 to 3 hours) because of their content of amorphous semilente insulin, but produce a smooth hypoglycaemic effect lasting up to 20 to 30 hours. They are much used, often in association with soluble insulin to provide a more rapid onset of action. Protamine zinc insulin has the longest duration of action because active insulin is only slowly released from the complex. It begins to work within 3 to 6 hours, but if used alone as a single morning injection it frequently causes hypoglycaemia during the early hours of the next morning. It is inadvisable to mix soluble and protamine zinc insulins in the same syringe because the latter contains excess protamine which will convert a proportion of the soluble insulin into long-acting insulin, and occasionally may lead to hyperglycaemia in the early stages and prolonged hypoglycaemia during the night.

Indications for use

Insulin is not needed in the majority of diabetics, who can be controlled on a low carbohydrate diet, either alone or in combination with oral therapy. However, in certain circumstances insulin is essential:

(a) In juvenile-onset diabetes.

(b) In maturity-onset diabetes which has not responded adequately to dietary control and oral hypoglycaemic drugs.

(c) In the patient presenting with diabetic coma.

(d) During intercurrent illness or surgery in patients who were formerly stable on diet or oral drugs.

(e) During pregnancy.

Initial stabilization of a patient on insulin is most easily performed using a sliding scale, by which the dosage is determined by the blood sugar level. Estimations are performed at 6 hourly intervals, and the dose is given as soluble insulin when the result is known. This scheme is suitable for the patient temporarily on insulin during surgery or an intercurrent illness. When control is satisfactory, it is sufficient to judge the dose of insulin by the amount of reducing substances in a sample of urine, as determined by 'Clinitest' tablets.

Once stabilization has been achieved, a trial of oral hypoglycaemic drugs is indicated in those patients whose daily requirement of insulin is low. This is unlikely to be successful, however, in a young patient, or in one who presented in diabetic coma. Where long-term insulin treatment is going to be necessary the soluble insulin should be replaced partly or entirely by a longer-acting preparation so that the frequency of administration is reduced. A mixture of soluble insulin and a long-acting preparation need be given only once a day for adequate control in many patients. Insulins are available in concentrations of 80, 40 and 20 (soluble only) units/ml, and the appropriate strength should be chosen to give a convenient volume for injection.

Diabetic ketoacidosis

Diabetic ketoacidosis and coma require urgent treatment with saline, potassium and insulin. Saline is given intravenously in large quantities because the patient is usually severely dehydrated. Potassium is added to the drip when the serum potassium falls to 4·5 mmol or less (potassium is drawn into the cells as the blood sugar falls and the acidosis is corrected). Soluble insulin is given in small doses, about 6 units/hour, by continuous intravenous infusion or by hourly intramuscular injection. Higher doses are necessary when the blood sugar response is not satisfactory, and this may be the case in the presence of an infection or if the patient has had steroids. When the blood sugar has fallen to 10 mmol, the insulin rate is halved and glucose is added to the infusion. When the patient is eating he is transferred to a twice daily insulin regime.

Adverse effects

The commonest adverse effect is hypoglycaemia, particularly at night with the long-acting preparations. Patients regularly receiving insulin soon get to know the warning symptoms and can counter it by taking sugar. Diabetics usually carry a card stating their condition and insulin requirements.

Areas of fat necrosis can occur in sites used repeatedly for injection, and can impair absorption. It may become necessary to use an alternative site. This, as mentioned above, is related to the immunogenicity of the preparation, and is greatest with standard beef insulins.

Oral hypoglycaemic drugs

Sulphonylureas

A chance observation that sulphonamide derivatives can lower the blood sugar led to the development of the sulphonylureas. Tolbutamide was the first clinically-useful drug, and this has been followed by chlorpropamide, acetohexamide, tolazamide, glibenclamide, glipizide and glibornuride. Glymidine is a closely related compound.

The hypoglycaemic effect of these compounds depends upon the presence of some functioning islet cells in the pancreas, for their chief mode of action is to promote insulin release. Nevertheless, they may also have peripheral actions, such as potentiating the tissue effects of insulin, reducing pancreatic glucagon secretion or decreasing the activity of hepatic insulinase.

Tolbutamide is rapidly carboxylated in the liver and therefore has a relatively short duration of action. It is usually administered three times daily.

Chlorpropamide is almost entirely excreted unchanged by the kidney and has a much longer half-life in the body (about 36 hours). It can exert a hypoglycaemic effect up to 10 days after its regular administration is stopped. It is given as a single daily dose.

The other sulphonylurea drugs are satisfactory alternatives to the above two, and can be useful when intolerance has developed to one of them. Glibenclamide is the most recent of these compounds, and resembles chlorpropamide in its duration of action. Weight for weight it is much more potent.

Adverse effects. The commonest adverse effects are urticarial skin lesions, leucopenia, nausea, vomiting, diarrhoea and constipation. Cholestatic jaundice occurs occasionally. Alcohol intolerance, characterized by facial flushing, may result from altered metabolism of alcohol, and is commoner with chlorpropamide. Changes in the protein-bound iodine level and the tri-iodothyronine resin uptake test have been shown to be produced by these drugs, but in the absence of clinical signs of hypothyroidism.

Hypoglycaemia is an important adverse effect, particularly in the elderly, in whom poor renal function can lead to accumulation of chlorpropamide. Profound hypoglycaemia, usually occurring at night, can produce permanent cerebral damage or death. For this reason the use of tolbutamide, rather than chlorpropamide, is preferable in elderly patients.

Sulphonylureas are strongly bound to plasma proteins, and this can lead to interactions with other drugs by competition for the same binding sites.

Biguanides

There are two important members of this group, metformin and phenformin. The use of the latter has been associated with lactic acidosis, sometimes fatal, and therefore metformin is to be preferred. Unlike the sulphonylureas, they do not promote insulin release from the pancreas. Their effect is a peripheral one but dependent upon the presence of circulating insulin. An effect on tissue enzymes responsible for glucose metabolism is their probable mechanism of action. This promotes peripheral uptake of both glucose and insulin. They do not produce hypoglycaemia in non-diabetic subjects. Postprandial hyperglycaemia and the subsequent rebound hypoglycaemia, which are often prediabetic signs in obese maturity-onset diabetics, are reduced by the biguanides.

Both metformin and phenformin are excreted unchanged by the kidneys, although phenformin is also partly metabolized in the liver. Phenformin has a slightly shorter duration of action (6 to 8 hours) than metformin (8 to 12 hours), but a slow-release preparation of phenformin is available, reducing the frequency of administration and producing a smoother action.

Adverse effects. The chief side-effects are anorexia, nausea, vomiting, and diarrhoea, and may be so troublesome that treatment has to be abandoned, and a sulphonylurea substituted.

Phenformin increases fibrinolytic activity, especially when combined with an anabolic steroid, and it reduces cholesterol synthesis.

Therapeutic use has been made of these effects, although the role of such treatment is uncertain.

Indications for use of oral hypoglycaemics

Dietary control of diabetes is the most important measure, and use of an oral hypoglycaemic drug is no substitute. Diet alone will control from 25 to 40 per cent of diabetic patients. A similar proportion require addition of an oral hypoglycaemic agent to achieve adequate control, while about 30 per cent will require insulin and diet.

Oral therapy is most appropriate in maturity-onset diabetics who have not been controlled by diet alone, who often have high levels of circulating insulin, and who show little tendency to develop ketosis. Biguanides are preferable to sulphonylureas in the markedly overweight patient, for the latter drugs cause an increase in weight, whereas the biguanides have an anorectic effect. When control is inadequate with one type of oral hypoglycaemic drug, combined sulphonylurea–biguanide treatment may be useful. The effects of each type of drug are additive, for they have a different mode of action. About 5 to 10 per cent of patients showing a good initial response to a sulphonylurea subsequently become inadequately controlled, and in these cases addition of a biguanide is valuable.

The place of oral hypoglycaemics in the management of young diabetics is strictly limited. They are occasionally used in children showing a period of amelioration of the symptoms soon after initial stabilization, but this is usually a temporary state of affairs and insulin is eventually required. Biguanides can be used as supplementary treatment in young diabetics with a high and fluctuating insulin requirement (the 'brittle' diabetic). In these patients the requirement may be reduced and made more stable. Oral therapy should be replaced by insulin during pregnancy, surgery, intercurrent infection or ketosis.

Oral hypoglycaemic drugs have an obvious advantage over insulin in the elderly and in those with failing sight. It is important, however, not to persist with oral therapy when control is inadequate. It should be remembered that renal function is usually reduced in the elderly, and this can lead to nocturnal hypoglycaemia with chlorpropamide.

Long-term effects of treatment

Whether rigorous control of the blood sugar level in diabetic patients reduces the incidence of subsequent complications of the disease is still uncertain. A study in the United States comparing the incidence of complications in patients treated with diet plus placebo, tolbutamide, phenformin or insulin, showed a significantly higher incidence of cardiovascular complications in patients receiving either of the two oral hypoglycaemics compared with patients on placebo or insulin. This study, however, has been criticized on several grounds, and the evidence which it provides does not, at this stage, condemn the use of oral drugs. Nevertheless, it underlines the prime importance of strict dietary control. Careful consideration should be given whenever the use of oral therapy is contemplated.

15

Drugs in endocrinology

THE HYPOTHALAMUS AND PITUITARY

The pituitary is responsible for the secretion of a number of important hormones, but is dependent upon the integrity of the hypothalamus to carry out this function. The posterior pituitary develops embryologically as an outgrowth from the brain, and remains connected to the hypothalamus by two important tracts of nerve fibres which act as channels down which the two posterior pituitary hormones are transported. The supraoptic nucleus situated above the optic chiasma in the hypothalamus produces vasopressin (antidiuretic hormone, ADH) which is transported down the supraoptico-hypophyseal tract to the pituitary, where it is released as needed from the nerve terminals. Oxytocin is produced in the paraventricular nucleus and is released from the pituitary in the same way. The connections are illustrated in Figure 17.

The anterior pituitary is derived from the foregut, not the brain, and is not connected to the hypothalamus by nervous pathways. Instead, a portal circulation develops which carries venous blood containing polypeptide hormones known as 'releasing factors' from the hypothalamus to a second capillary bed in the anterior pituitary. These factors liberate the anterior pituitary hormones from their granular stores. Releasing hormones have been described for thyroid-stimulating hormone (TSH), the gonadotrophins (follicle-stimulating hormone, FSH, and luteinizing hormone, LH), prolactin, adrenocorticotrophin (ACTH) and melanocyte-stimulating hormone (MSH). The structures of two of the releasing hormones, thyrotrophin-releasing hormone (TRH) and gonadotrophin-releasing hormone (LH/FSH-RH), are known.

The release of two hormones, prolactin and growth hormone (GH), and possibly a third, MSH, are also controlled by release-inhibiting hormones. The structure of growth hormone release-inhibiting hormone is known. Dopamine may be the prolactin release-inhibiting factor. Drugs which impair dopaminergic transmission, such as phenothiazines, reserpine, α-methyl dopa and metoclopramide, can cause hyperprolactinaemia and galactorrhoea by impairing the inhibitory control of prolactin release.

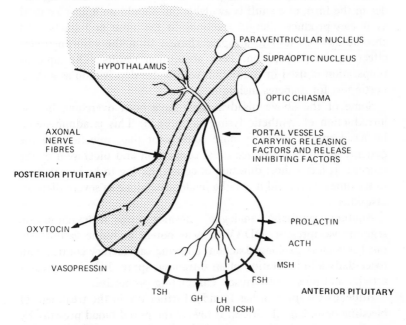

Fig. 17 Mechanisms controlling the secretion of pituitary hormones.

POSTERIOR PITUITARY HORMONES

Vasopressin (ADH)

In physiological amounts vasopressin acts on the distal and collecting tubules of the kidney, increasing their permeability to water and thereby conserving water. The absence of this hormone produces diabetes insipidus. This occurs as a permanent feature only when the supraoptic region of the hypothalamus is destroyed. Posterior pituitary damage causes only temporary derangement of vasopressin secretion. In larger doses the hormone produces a pressor response by peripheral vasoconstriction, angina from coronary vasoconstriction, and abdominal colic.

For clinical use vasopressin is available as pitressin of pig or beef origin, or in the synthetic forms of lysine-vasopressin (LVP) or desmopressin. Pitressin of animal origin is usually administered as pitressin tannate in oil, which acts for a longer time than aqueous solutions and is suitable for long term management of diabetes insipidus. It needs to be given intramuscularly every 1 to 3 days. Repeated injection into the same area of skin can lead to accumulation of oil and impaired absorption of the hormone. Pitressin powder in the form of a snuff is available but should no longer be used as it can produce allergic reactions in the nose and lungs, and chronic use can lead to atrophic rhinitis from the vasoconstrictor effect of the preparation. Poor absorption results. The aqueous preparation is used in conjuction with water deprivation as a diagnostic test for diabetes insipidus.

Some of the above disadvantages have been overcome by the introduction of synthetic lysine vasopressin. This is administered by nasal spray, which is more convenient than injection for the patient, but it can produce nasal congestion and ulceration of the mucosa. It has a short duration of action, having to be repeated up to six times daily, and it may be inadequate alone in severe diabetes insipidus.

Another synthetic analogue, desmopressin (I-desamino-8-D-arginine vasopressin, DDAVP), is as potent as lysine vasopressin but has a more prolonged action, allowing satisfactory control with twice-daily administration of an intranasal spray. It has no pressor activity and no smooth muscle contracting properties.

Aqueous vasopressin has found a further use in the treatment of bleeding oesophageal varices. It lowers the portal blood pressure by producing splanchnic vasoconstriction, and thus the bleeding from anastomotic vessels is reduced. It also promotes the passage of blood clot through the intestine, reducing the likelihood of hepatic coma from digestion of blood proteins.

Treatment of diabetes insipidus. Although vasopressin is the mainstay of treatment, oral agents have been sought because of their convenience. Sulphonylureas, particularly chlorpropamide, reduce polyuria in hypothalamic diabetes insipidus, but not in the nephrogenic form of the disease, which is caused by renal insensitivity to the circulating hormone. They sensitize the renal tubules to diminished amounts of circulating vasopressin, but are ineffective when there is a complete absence of the hormone, e.g. post-hypophysectomy. Chlorpropamide requires about three days to produce its effect. It can control mild diabetes insipidus when given alone, but in more severe disease the addition of vasopressin is necessary. Dilutional hyponatraemia can occur if the level of circulating vasopressin is fluctuating, or if chlorpropamide and vasopressin are given together without water restriction. Hypoglycaemia may also occur. Thiazide diuretics are less effective than chlorpropamide in hypothalamic diabetes insipidus, but unlike the latter drug they have a clinically useful effect in the nephrogenic type, especially if sodium intake is restricted at the same time. Oral potassium supplements are necessary to avoid hypokalaemia.

Oxytocin

Oxytocin causes a contraction of uterine smooth muscle, the sensitivity of which gradually increases during pregnancy. Although the role of this hormone during normal labour is not clear, when given by intravenous infusion it induces labour, and is widely used for this purpose. Dangerously powerful contractions can be produced by excessive doses. Oxytocin is released by stimulation of afferent fibres of the lactating breast, and it causes contraction of the myoepithelial cells with ejection of milk. This accounts for the uterine contractions which accompany breast-feeding postpartum. Oxytocin is usually given in a synthetic form, although an extract of mammalian pituitary glands is still available.

Other drugs acting on the uterus

Ergometrine. It is now standard procedure in obstetric practice to administer intramuscular ergometrine on the crowning of the foetal head. By the time the placenta has been delivered the drug is producing its effect. Ergometrine has a direct stimulant action on the uterine muscle, causing a rapid contraction of the uterus and a reduced incidence of postpartum haemorrhage. Ergotamine also stimulates the uterus, but its more powerful peripheral vasoconstrictor action makes it less suitable for obstetric use. In addition to their direct effects on smooth muscle both drugs have an α-adrenolytic activity, but this is of no therapeutic value. A preparation (Syntometrine) combining synthetic oxytocin and ergometrine is available, and produces more rapid contraction of the uterus than ergometrine alone.

Prostaglandins. Amongst their many actions prostaglandins of the E and F series stimulate the myometrium. Their presence in human seminal, menstrual and amniotic fluids, and in the maternal circulation during labour and abortion, suggests that they may have an important role in uterine function during conception and labour. Prostaglandins E_2 and $F_{2\alpha}$ are widely used both orally and by intravenous infusion for induction of labour and abortion, and are given to promote cervical ripening. Prostaglandin $F_{2\alpha}$ produces more side-effects, notably nausea, vomiting and diarrhoea.

Non-steroidal anti-inflammatory drugs. By inhibiting prostaglandin synthesis, aspirin and other anti-inflammatory drugs inhibit uterine motility and have therefore been used to inhibit preterm labour. Unfortunately, they can cross the placental barrier and can cause premature closure of the ductus arteriosus, leading to primary pulmonary hypertension of the newborn. They are therefore contraindicated in pregnancy and labour. Non-steroidal anti-inflammatory drugs are being used in patent-ductus arteriosus in neonates (p. 136).

Sympathomimetic drugs. Stimulation of β-adrenergic receptors in the uterus produces relaxation of the myometrium. Isoxsuprine, ritodrine orciprenaline and salbutamol, all having predominant β_2-mimetic activity, are of value in arresting premature labour.

ANTERIOR PITUITARY HORMONES

Growth hormone

Growth hormone has several functions, (a) it promotes longitudinal growth of long bones, (b) it is concerned in the growth and maturation of the viscera and soft tissues, (c) it elevates the blood glucose level by anti-insulin action, and (d) it stimulates protein synthesis and fat breakdown. Its effects on bone growth are dependent upon the levels of circulating sex hormones, for the latter are responsible for bone maturation and fusion of the epiphyses, and growth hormone can only produce lengthening when the epiphyses are unfused. Thus an excess of growth hormone with normal levels of sex hormones during childhood produces gigantism, whereas in adults it will lead to the clinical features of acromegaly. A deficiency of growth hormone in childhood produces patients of short stature and with delayed puberty, although they eventually become fertile. It is important to institute replacement therapy at the earliest opportunity in these children.

Growth hormone is a polypeptide comprising 188 amino acids. It has not been synthesized, and because of species differences in structure, growth hormone obtained from any source other than man or monkey is of no value in treating patients. In the United Kingdom human growth hormone is extracted from pituitary glands collected at post-mortem by pathologists throughout the country, and is distributed by the Medical Research Council. Because supplies are limited there are strict criteria laid down which have to be satisfied before a patient qualifies for treatment. It is given intramuscularly two or three times weekly, and is effective in stimulating growth in children whose small stature is due to growth hormone deficiency, but in other types of dwarfism response is disappointing.

Growth-hormone release-inhibiting hormone (GH-RIH, somatostatin), whose structure has been characterized, regulates the pituitary release of growth hormone. Development of a long-acting preparation should prove a major advance in the treatment of acromegaly. It also reduces insulin and glucagon secretion by a direct action on the pancreas, which may be of future therapeutic value.

The semi-synthetic ergot alkaloid, bromocriptine (α-bromo ergocriptine) reduces elevated growth hormone levels and relieves the symptoms of acromegaly. It has been an important advance in the management of this condition. It stimulates dopamine receptors in the CNS.

Prolactin
Raised levels of circulating prolactin have been demonstrated in patients with galactorrhoea from a variety of causes, among which are a number of drugs, including phenothiazines, metoclopramide, reserpine, imipramine, haloperidol, α-methyl dopa and oral contraceptives. All but the last of these impair dopaminergic transmission, which account for their ability to produce this effect. As the secretion of prolactin from the pituitary is held in check by a hypothalamic inhibitory factor, probably dopamine, galactorrhoea is the result of a suppression of the release of this factor or by blockade of its effects on the pituitary.

The dopamine agonist drug, bromocriptine, reduces raised serum prolactin levels and is used in treating galactorrhoea associated with amenorrhea. Galactorrhoea responds rapidly and normal menstrual periods are restored within a few weeks. Bromocriptine can be used in the presence of a pituitary tumour. In amenorrhoeic patients with a normal prolactin level, no response is seen. Its dopamine agonist properties probably explain its therapeutic effect.

Gonadotrophins
Antibodies are quickly developed to gonadotrophins of animal origin so human material has to be used in treating gonadotrophin deficiency. Although they can be extracted from pituitary glands, human menopausal urinary gonadrotrophin (HMG) is rich in FSH and LH and this is the usual source of these hormones. Human chorionic gonadotrophin (HCG), obtained from the urine of pregnant women, has actions similar to those of LH and is often used in conjunction with HMG.

Gonadotrophin deficiency causes delayed puberty in children, impotence and infertility in adult males, and oligo- or amenorrhoea with infertility in women. In order to promote ovulation in women HMG is given until an ovarian response has been detected, as judged by clinical signs of oestrogenic effects and by increasing levels of urinary oestrogen, and then HCG is given to induce ovulation. Infertility from causes other than gonadotrophin deficiency does not respond to this treatment. In males HCG has the same effect as ICSH (LH) and can be used to stimulate testosterone production from the interstitial cells, which leads to the development of secondary sexual characteristics in patients with delayed puberty. Spermatogenesis is stimulated by HMG, but prolonged treatment is required, sometimes with ICSH supplements.

Clomiphene. Clomiphene is a gonadotrophin-releasing agent, acting by blocking the negative feedback receptor sites in the hypothalamus. It is used in the diagnosis and treatment of hypogonadism and infertility. In patients who have low circulating levels of gonadotrophins a failure to increase these levels after administration of clomiphene suggests a hypothalamic-pituitary cause. Treatment with clomiphene can often induce ovulation in infertile hypo- or normogonadotrophic women.

Thyroid stimulating hormone
TSH stimulates the uptake of iodine by the thyroid gland and promotes release of thyroxine and triiodothyronine. It is used diagnostically in hypothyroidism to distinguish intrinsic thyroid disease from a disorder of hypothalamic–pituitary function. When the thyroid gland is normal, TSH will cause a release of thyroid hormones. It is also of value for assessing thyroid function in patients already receiving thyroxine, or in identifying metastases from a

Adrenocorticotrophic hormone (see page 205)

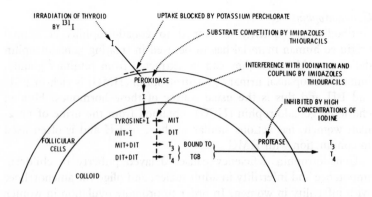

Fig. 18 Synthesis of thyroid hormones and its modification by antithyroid drugs.

thyroid carcinoma, for it promotes uptake of radio-iodine, which can be assessed by scanning. TSH is of bovine origin, and allergic reactions to it can occur.

Thyrotrophin-releasing hormone (TRH), whose structure has been elucidated, can be used diagnostically to distinguish between primary hypothyroidism and that secondary to pituitary disease.

THYROID HORMONES

The thyroid gland secretes a mixture of thyroxine (T_4) and tri-iodothyronine (T_3) in the ratio of 50:1. They are synthesized in the thyroid gland by iodination of tyrosine, forming mono- and diiodotyrosine, which subsequently conjugate to form T_3 and T_4 (Fig. 18). All these reactions occur while the constituents are bound to thyroglobulin, and the hormones have to be split off by a protease enzyme before they can enter the circulation. T_3 is about four times more potent than T_4 in increasing the metabolic rate, and thus both hormones contribute to the metabolic effects produced by thyroid secretions. In hyperthyroidism there is usually an increase in both hormones, but occasionally only the T_3 fraction is elevated.

Treatment of hypothyroidism

T_4 is usually used for replacement therapy. There is seldom an indication for giving T_3. Thyroid extract, prepared from pork or beef thyroid glands, contains both hormones, but this preparation is poorly standardized and therefore variable in its effects. As T_4 can be synthesized and precisely standardized, it has rendered thyroid extract obsolete.

Synthetic T_4 is the sodium salt of L-thyroxine. For full replacement 200 to 300 μg daily are required. One to two weeks is required for its effects to become maximal, and they persist for several weeks after discontinuing treatment. The reason for this is that T_4 is about 99·9 per cent protein bound in serum and tissues, so it takes some days to saturate these physiologically-inactive stores. Caution should be exercised in administering the drug to the elderly or those with ischaemic heart disease, in whom angina of effort or heart failure can be precipitated. The dose should be increased cautiously, and rarely needs to be greater than 200 μg daily. Addition of a β-adrenergic blocker may reduce the occurrence of angina. Monitoring the serum TSH level will assist in tailoring the dosage to suit the patient; the level will fall to normal when the optimum dose has been achieved.

Liothyronine is the sodium salt of triiodothyronine. Being less protein bound it acts more quickly than T₄, the peak effect occurring about 48 hours after a single dose. There are two indications for its use in preference to T₄, (a) in the treatment of myxoedema coma, and (b) when it is necessary to stop treatment from time to time to perform scanning studies, e.g. in looking for secondaries after surgical treatment of a thyroid carcinoma.

For the treatment of myxoedema coma it is usual to give 10 to 20   μg of T₃ and 50 mg of hydrocortisone hemisuccinate intravenously every 12 hours initially, but oral administration of T₄ should begin as soon as possible. Administration of hydrocortisone is of utmost importance as prolonged hypothyroidism usually depresses adrenocortical function, and the increase in metabolic activity produced by T₃ puts immediate demands on this.

Treatment of hyperthyroidism

The object of treatment is to reduce the synthesis and release of thyroid hormones. This can be done in several ways, as are summarized in Figure 18.

Potassium perchlorate. Uptake of iodine is blocked by this drug, but the block can be overcome by a modest intake of iodine, e.g. in a cough mixture. Agranulocytosis and fatal aplastic anaemia occur rarely, but with sufficient frequency for its use to be reserved for those patients who cannot tolerate an imidazole or thiouracil derivative.

Imidazoles. Carbimazole is the drug of first choice. It inhibits, by substrate competition, the peroxidase enzyme which releases iodine from circulating iodides, and, in addition, it inhibits the enzymes responsible for iodination of tyrosine and coupling of the iodinated derivatives. It is suitable for use in most types of hyperthyroidism where drug therapy is preferred to surgery or radioiodine treatment. The starting dose is chosen according to the severity of the disease. The object is to render the patient euthyroid and then to reduce to a maintenance dose. Concurrent administration of T₄ prevents hypothyroidism and avoids difficulty in dose titration. Withdrawal of the drug is often possible after one to two years, although relapse occurs in a proportion of patients.

Methimazole is similar.

Hypothyroidism and enlargement of the thyroid can occur with excessive doses of an imidazole. Rashes occur often, and agranulocytosis is seen occasionally.

Thiouracils. Propyl- and methylthiouracil have actions resembling those of the imidazoles. They are usually reserved for those patients who are intolerant of the latter drugs.

Iodine and iodides. In pharmacological doses iodine or potassium iodide cause inhibition of the release of T_3 and T_4 from the colloidal stores of the thyroid gland. Their use is reserved for the preoperative preparation of patients for thyroidectomy, because the vascularity of the gland is reduced by these compounds. The effect is transient and therefore the operation should be performed 2 to 3 weeks after starting treatment. In other than mild cases previous treatment with a thiouracil or imidazole is necessary. Iodine should not be given immediately after treatment with potassium perchlorate, for it can produce a thyroid crisis by sudden release of hormones. Iodine or iodine-containing medicines (e.g. cough mixtures) taken during pregnancy can cause a goitre in the foetus.

Radioactive iodine. Because iodine is concentrated in the thyroid gland, a small dose of radioactive iodine will irradiate the hormone-producing follicular cells. [131]I has been widely used for this purpose, and is a valuable alternative to surgery. It should not be used in children or in women of childbearing age. One of the chief disadvantages of this treatment is the frequency with which postirradiation hypothyroidism occurs. For this reason ^{125}I is undergoing trials. In theory this isotope might be preferable because its emission is less penetrating than that of ^{131}I, and should cause less damage to the nuclei of the follicular cells, but assessment of its possible advantages must await the results of long-term follow-up in these trials.

Adrenergic-blocking drugs. β-Receptor blocking drugs can reduce the heart rate and peripheral manifestations of hyperthyroidism, and can therefore be useful as an adjunct to treatment with antithyroid drugs. Blocking drugs without intrinsic sympathomimetic properties, such as propranolol, are preferable. Heart failure is not an absolute contraindication to propranolol so long as vigorous treatment with digoxin and diuretics is started simultaneously.

Treatment of exophthalmos

In some patients with hyperthyroidism, exophthalmos is troubling or even threatening to the eyes. Unfortunately, it usually does not respond to treatment of the hyperthyroid state, although the accompanying lid retraction is reduced. The levator palpebrae is partly composed of adrenergically innervated smooth muscle, and the adrenergic nerve blocking drug guanethidine usually relieves lid retraction when instilled into the lacrymal sac. Unfortunately, it often aggravates the grittiness of the conjunctiva which occurs in the exophthalmic eye. Methylcellulose drops can help by lubricating the conjunctiva and lids. In severe cases corticosteroids or surgical decompression of the orbit is necessary.

Parathyroid hormone and calcitonin

The principle physiological function of parathyroid hormone is to maintain a normal plasma calcium level. It does so probably by effects on bone metabolism, and on the renal excretion and intestinal absorption of calcium. These effects are closely interrelated with the tissue effects of vitamin D. A parenteral preparation containing parathyroid extract is available and is used diagnostically as well as in the treatment of tetany. It is too antigenic for long-term use in hypoparathyroidism, the management of which depends upon administration of vitamin D or dihydrotachysterol (see p. 215).

The normal physiological role of calcitonin is uncertain, but it is capable of reducing elevated calcium levels. Preparations are available containing either porcine or synthetic salmon calcitonin. The latter is less antigenic and is proving useful in inhibiting the excessive bone resorption and relieving bone pain in Paget's disease, and in the management of severe hypercalcaemia.

SEX HORMONES

Androgens and anabolic steroids

Androgens have two main types of action, (a) development of the secondary sexual characteristics of the male and growth of the genitalia, and (b) anabolic effects, such as retention of nitrogen, synthesis of body proteins, development of the musculature and bones, and fusion of the epiphyses. It has been possible to separate partly these effects so that some compounds have predominant anabolic actions, and although they are widely used in patients with chronic debilitating diseases the evidence that they promote recovery is conflicting.

Androgenic preparations

Testosterone is the chief androgen secreted by the testes and adrenal cortex under the pituitary control of ICSH. Testosterone is converted to its active metabolite, 5-α-dihydrotestosterone, in the target cells. A deficiency of this hormone starting in childhood produces eunuchoidism, but when it starts after puberty it causes a regression of secondary sexual characteristics, loss of libido and infertility. Testosterone is used for replacement therapy, but the

unmodified molecule is rapidly metabolized. Esterification length
ens the duration of action. It can be given in a number of ways,
sublingually as testosterone propionate in a waxy base, intramuscularly as the propionate in water or oenanthate in oil, or by subcutaneous implantation as testosterone pellets. Flumesterone, a
synthetic androgen, can be given orally. Methyltestosterone is
available for sublingual administration, but it is poorly absorbed
and occasionally causes cholestatic jaundice.

Indication for use of androgens
(a) *Replacement therapy in hypogonadism.* Testosterone will induce
sexual development when puberty is delayed, and will restore
potency and libido in adults who have developed androgen deficiency, regardless of whether it is due to testicular or pituitary disorder. When the deficiency is secondary to pituitary disease, however, it is preferable to use HCG to induce puberty. Fertility can be
restored only if the seminiferous tubules of the testes are functional, and are stimulated by administration of gonadotrophins.
   (b) *Growth disorders.* Growth can be curtailed by stimulating
epiphyseal fusion in boys growing to an excessive height. Although
an initial growth spurt is produced in dwarfism, early fusion of the
epiphyses can cause greater curtailment of growth than would have
occurred in the absence of treatment, especially if used in excessive
dosage.

Anabolic steroids
A number of these are available, the more important being nan-
drolone, methanolone, methandienone and norethandrolone. These
compounds are used to encourage protein anabolism in chronic disease, following major surgery or in patients with 'senile'
osteoporosis, but there is no good evidence as yet that they are of
real value. Their ability to reduce protein catabolism is used to
delay uraemia in patients with acute renal failure. Androgens or
anabolic steroids are sometimes of value in inhibiting the growth of
a breast carcinoma, particularly in premenopausal women, and in
the management of aplastic anaemia. Oxymethalone is the drug of
choice in the latter. Although anabolic steroids have less marked
androgenic properties than testosterone, they can cause masculinization in women. They will also cause masculinization of the
foetus if used during pregnancy.

Oestrogens
Oestrogens are produced mainly in the ovary and placenta, but

small amounts are synthesized in the adrenal and testes. The three important oestrogens are oestrone, oestradiol and oestriol. The last of these is a physiologically active metabolite of oestradiol, and is produced in large quantities by the placenta. Its main effects are on the cervix and vaginal epithelium, while oestradiol influences endometrial development.

For therapeutic use oestrogens can be given in a variety of forms, but essentially these can be divided into two classes, (a) naturally occurring steroid hormones or their derivatives, and (b) synthetic non-steroid compounds with oestrogenic effects.

Steroid hormones and derivatives. Naturally-occurring hormones have a rather short-lived effect because they are metabolized quickly. A number of derivatives of oestradiol have been produced and these form the basis of many preparations. Two orally-active derivatives, ethinyloestradiol and mestranol, are widely used, and most combined oestrogen-progestogen contraceptive pills are based on these two oestrogens. Oestradiol monobenzoate is a longer acting parenteral preparation which is slowly hydrolyzed to release oestradiol. Oestradiol valerate can be injected as an oily solution from which it is slowly absorbed.

One proprietary preparation, Premarin, contains natural oestrogens, equilin and equilenin, which are extracted from mare's urine.

Non-steroid oestrogens. Stilboestrol is the most important of these and is active orally. Alternative drugs are dienoestrol, methallenoestril, and chlorotrianisene.

Indications for oestrogen therapy

(a) Menorrhagia can be controlled by administration of oestrogens in high dosage, but a gradual tailing-off is necessary if withdrawal bleeding is not to be precipitated. This problem, however, has been largely overcome by the use of oestrogen-progestogen combinations, for the progestogen produces secretory changes in the endometrum which prevent severe bleeding. High doses of oestrogens can cause nausea.

(b) Climacteric symptoms respond to oestrogen treatment, but often at the expense of some degree of post menopausal bleeding. Oestriol produces little or no bleeding. Oestrogens prevent excess bone loss following premature menopause.

(c) Amenorrhoea is usually caused by hypothalamic–pituitary disorder rather than ovarian disease, and oestrogen-withdrawal bleeding can usually be induced. Accompanying underdevelopment of secondary sexual characteristics will respond to oestrogen administration, but infertility will not. Gonadotrophin or clomi-phene treatment is necessary to induce ovulation. Oligomenor-rhoea may be worsened by oestrogen treatment, which can further disrupt the pituitary-ovarian feedback mechanism.

(d) Endometriosis can often be cured by prolonged use of oestrogen-progestogen combinations, but the use of progesterone preparations alone is found satisfactory by some. The aim is to produce atrophy of the ectopic endometrial tissue.

(e) The use of stilboestrol in the treatment of threatened abor-tion has been discontinued since it was recognized that vaginal adenocarcinoma could occur in the adolescent daughters of mothers treated with the drug.

(f) Lactation can be suppressed in mothers who do not wish to breast feed. Bromocriptine is preferable to oestrogens for this pur-pose, however, because it specifically reduces prolactin levels by acting on the pituitary. However, in practice simpler methods usually suffice e.g. avoiding nipple stimulation and breast support.

(g) Carcinoma of the prostate often responds dramatically to oes-trogen therapy, but feminization and thrombo-embolic disease can be produced.

Progestogens

Progesterone is produced naturally by the corpus luteum and placenta, and it has two main functions, (a) to induce secretory changes in the endometrium in the luteal phase of the menstrual cycle, and (b) to maintain pregnancy after implantation of the ovum. Progestogens are used therapeutically to encourage these effects when natural control seems to be lacking.

Progesterone itself is very insoluble and has a short half-life in the body. Although it can be given in oil, synthetic substitutes are preferable. These are derived from two steroid substances, nortes-tosterone and 17α-hydroxyprogesterone. Nortestosterone is derived from testosterone by demethylation, and from it are pro-duced the most-used synthetic progestogens, norethisterone, norethynodrel, lynestrenol and ethynodiol. These compounds have marked progestogenic effects, but, with the exception of allyles-trenol, they retain slight androgenic properties which make them unsuitable for use during early pregnancy, because they can have a virilizing effect in the foetus. In the adult female, however, these effects are negligible. They are metabolized to a small extent to oestrogenic substances, which give them oestrogenic properties in addition. However, they are usually administered in combination with oestrogens in order to suppress ovulation for contraceptive purposes and for the treatment of menstrual disorders.

17α-Hydroxyprogesterone is an intermediate in the biosynthesis of cortisol, but is not secreted as a progestogen by the adrenal cortex. Esterification of this compound yields megestrol acetate, which has a negligible oestrogenic or androgenic effect, and is suitable for use in pregnant women.

Indications for progestogen therapy
(a) *Menstrual disorders.* A combination of oestrogen and progestogen will impose a regular menstrual pattern in most cases of menorrhagia and metrorrhagia. Dysmenorrhoea often disappears, and endometriosis can be cured by long-term use of these combinations. Symptoms of premenstrual tension often respond to non-oestrogenic progestogens given alone. Bromocriptine is known to reduce breast discomfort, but its role in treatment is uncertain.

(b) *To prevent abortion.* Progestogens are still widely used for preventing threatened abortion or premature labour, although it is likely that they are of value only when there is a deficiency of maternal progestogens. Allylestrenol is to be preferred because it is non-virilizing.

(c) *Carcinoma of the uterine body.* Progestogens are useful in treating metastases after the primary has been excised.

The contraceptive pill
The pills most widely used are combinations of a progestogen and an oestrogen (see Table 14). Only two oestrogenic compounds are used in the pill whereas a variety of progestogens have been used, synthesised either from 19-nortestosterone or from 17-α-hydroxyprogesterone. Derivatives of 19-nortestosterone are metabolised to a small extent to oestrogenic compounds, unlike the

Table 14 Oestrogens and progestogens used in the Pill

Oestrogens	Progestogens
Ethinyloestradiol	**Derivatives of 19-nortestosterone**
	Norethynodrel
Mestranol (3-methyl	Norethisterone
ether of	Ethynodiol diacetate
ethinyloestradiol)	Lynestrenol
	Norgestrel
	Derivatives of 17 α-hydroxyprogesterone
	Medroxyprogesterone acetate
	Megestrol acetate

17α-hydroxyprogesterone derivatives, and this may account for their powerful ovulation suppressant action. Most combination pills contain a 19-nortestosterone derivative plus an oestrogen.

Mode of action

The oestrogenic compounds ethinyloestradiol and mestranol suppress ovulation by inhibiting the release of FSH from the anterior pituitary. In combination with a progestogen, particularly a 19-nortestosterone derivative, the antiovulatory effect largely accounts for the contraceptive action. Other changes take place, however, and contribute to this action. For instance, pseudo-decidual reactions occur in the endometrium and implantation of a fertilized ovum is impaired. The secretion of cervical mucus is reduced and it becomes thick and viscous so that spermatozoa are less able to penetrate into the uterine cavity. Furthermore, it is possible that the function of the corpus luteum might be disturbed by 17 α-hydroxyprogesterone derivatives.

(a) *Progestogen-oestrogen combinations*. These are usually taken for 21 or 22 days of the menstrual cycle, starting on the fifth day (counting from the onset of menstruation). A tablet-free interval of 6 or 7 days is then allowed, making a 28-day cycle. Withdrawal bleeding occurs during the tablet-free interval.

(b) *Sequential pills*. These were developed in an attempt to achieve a more physiological control over ovulation. In the first part of the cycle, usually up to day 16 or 20, an oestrogen-only pill is taken, followed by a combined oestrogen-progestogen pill until day 25 or 26. A drug-free interval of 7 days is then allowed.

(c) *Low-dose progestogen-only pills*. Concern over the adverse effects of oestrogen therapy has stimulated the development of pills containing only a progestogen in low dosage which is taken continuously. The contraceptive action of these pills is more limited, and ovulation can occur in up to 40 per cent of cycles. Biochemical changes in cervical mucus probably account largely for the contraceptive action. This method cannot be recommended when a low failure rate is essential. Irregular menstrual bleeding is common.

Minor adverse effects

The following occur commonly on starting the pill:

(i) *Nausea and occasional vomiting* is common in the first cycle but usually settles in subsequent months. If it persists, a pregnancy test should be performed. Nausea is caused by the oestrogen component and a change to a less oestrogenic pill may help.

(ii) *Breast tenderness* and slight enlargement may occur during the first few cycles. It is an oestrogenic effect similar to that occurring in pregnancy.

(*iii*) *Weight gain* is common with some progestogenic preparations but is usually small and is lost after a few cycles.

(*iv*) *Break-through bleeding*, i.e. menstrual 'spotting' occurring in mid-cycle, is seen frequently at first especially with low-oestrogen pills and low-dose progestogen-only pills.

(*v*) *Post-pill amenorrhoea and hypofertility* may occur, and can sometimes be prolonged.

Serious adverse effects

These, fortunately, occur rarely:

(*i*) *Thrombo-embolic disease.* In the early 1960s, soon after the introduction of the contraceptive pill, reports began to appear of venous thrombo-embolism occurring in young women using the pill, and by 1966 a large number of case reports had appeared.

The results of formal epidemiological studies indicated that deep vein thrombosis and pulmonary embolism occurred more often than would be expected by chance alone in women taking the contraceptive pill. The relative risk was approximately 6–8 times greater in pill takers. The incidence correlates with both the dose of oestrogen and the dose of progestogen in the pill.

(*ii*) *Ischaemic cerebrovascular disorders.* The incidence of cerebral thrombosis is 5–6 times greater in women taking the pill. Cerebrovascular disease is normally rare in young women, which makes even more impressive the numbers of such cases reported in relationship to the contraceptive pill.

Assessment of the risk of thrombo-embolism associated with the use of the contraceptive pill requires consideration of a number of factors. The morbidity, and even the mortality, produced by other forms of contraception is not negligible and the risk of unwanted pregnancy may be higher than with the pill. Pregnancy itself causes an appreciable risk of complications, and legal abortion when unintended pregnancies occur is also not without hazard. It has been suggested that one oral contraceptive pill is as dangerous as smoking one-third of a cigarette once a day for three weeks out of four.

In 1970, the Committee on Safety of Medicines considered that the evidence incriminating the oestrogen component of the contraceptive pill was strong enough to recommend that preparations containing no more than 50 μg of oestrogen should be used. Since this recommendation, the dose has been further reduced to 30 or 20 μg in some preparations, and there is evidence that this lessens the incidence of thromboembolic disease further. Low-dose progestogen-only pills seemed to be associated with a low risk, whereas sequential preparations produced a high risk.

(*iii*) *Myocardial infarction.* The incidence of pill taking in young women admitted to coronary care units is considerably higher than the expected incidence. In some women aged 40 or more on the combined pill, the risk of death from infarction approaches the incidence in males of a similar age.

(*iv*) *Hypertension.* Blood pressure is on average significantly increased by the contraceptive pill. Several high risk factors have been identified, such as obesity, a past history of toxaemia of pregnancy, and a family history of hypertension.

(*v*) *Jaundice.* It is not surprising that oral contraceptives can cause jaundice, for many are 17α-alkyl-substituted steroids, and compounds of this type were known to be capable of causing cholestasis before the pill was introduced.

(*vi*) *Haemangioma of liver.* There is evidence of an increased incidence following long-term administration of the combined contraceptive pill.

Other adverse effects
The contraceptive pill has been held responsible for a number of other adverse effects, although in some cases the relationship has not been convincingly proven.

(*i*) *Depression, headaches and loss of libido* occur frequently, but it must be remembered that these symptoms are common and should not always be put down to the pill.

(*ii*) *Impairment of glucose tolerance* can be caused by an effect on peripheral glucose metabolism, and occurs particularly in women with a family history of diabetes. Pre-existing diabetes may be worsened.

(*iii*) *Fluid retention* can occur, and care should be taken when prescribing for patients with renal or cardiac disease.

(*iv*) *Intolerance to contact lenses* has been reported.

(*v*) *Carcinogenic effects* do not occur. In fact the incidence of some carcinomas, e.g. carcinoma of the cervix, may be reduced.

(*vi*) *Interactions* with the pill. These include interactions with liver enzyme inducers (see p. 23), and with broad-spectrum antibiotics such as amoxycillin which reduce their contraceptive effectiveness by interfering with enterohepatic cycling.

Conditions in which oestrogenic preparations should be avoided
A full medical examination is necessary before the pill is prescribed. Certain diseases are absolute contraindications to administration of oestrogenic preparations:

(i) Heart disease, and a previous history of thrombo-embolism. Caution may be necessary in a woman with hypertension.

(ii) Hepatic disease, including biliary cirrhosis, chronic active hepatitis, Dubin-Johnson and Rotor syndromes, and a history of idiopathic jaundice of pregnancy.

(iii) Cancers of the breast or genital tract.

(iv) Porphyria.

(v) Sickle cell anaemia.

16

Mild analgesics, anti-inflammatory drugs and corticosteroids

INFLAMMATION

The inflammatory reaction, both acute and chronic, is a basic defensive response to a variety of forms of injury. Some of the features of this reaction can be induced by a number of chemical mediators including kinins and histamine, but recent evidence suggests that prostaglandins may be of particular importance in many types of inflammation. They have been detected in exudates from experimentally induced inflammation, and abnormally high concentrations of prostaglandins E_1, E_2, $F_{1\alpha}$, and $F_{2\alpha}$ were found when perfusion studies were carried out in the skin lesions of allergic volunteers with contact dermatitis.

Several different classes of drug possess anti-inflammatory properties and it has been difficult to define a mechanism of action common to them all. There is increasing evidence, however, that many of them interfere with prostaglandin activity. For example, aspirin, sodium salicylate, indomethacin and corticosteroids, in therapeutic concentrations, inhibit the synthesis of prostaglandins E_2 and $F_{2\alpha}$ from arachidonic acid by animal tissues. Fenamic acids, phenylbutazone and aspirin block the bronchoconstrictor effects of prostaglandin $F_{2\alpha}$. It may be, therefore, that the anti-inflammatory drugs to be described possess in common the ability either to inhibit the synthesis or to block the activity of prostaglandins which mediate the inflammatory response.

In diseases in which inflammation is the cause of pain, e.g. rheumatoid arthritis, it is logical to choose an analgesic drug with powerful anti-inflammatory activity, although drugs lacking this effect will nevertheless give satisfactory pain relief in mild disease. Many of the available analgesics have a central component to their therapeutic effect, although the relative contribution of such an action to the total drug effect may be difficult to determine.

MILD ANALGESICS AND ANTI-INFLAMMATORY DRUGS

The range of mild analgesic and anti-inflammatory drugs available is now wide. Aspirin still has an important place and serves as a model drug with which to compare newer preparations.

Aspirin

Although salicylates occur naturally, aspirin (acetylsalicylic acid) is a synthetic substance, and remains the most popular of remedies for minor ailments, having displaced quinine from this position early in the present century. It is consumed in vast quantities and this vouches for its relative safety. It is available in many different forms and presentations, but in practical terms there is little to choose between them. Plain aspirin is the free acid, and is less soluble than its calcium salt ('soluble aspirin'). Aspirin can cause gastric bleeding, and it was thought that this was the result of erosion of the mucosa by a poorly soluble tablet sticking to it. Soluble aspirin, however, is no better in this respect, although it is absorbed more quickly. Aspirin is combined in a number of preparations with a variety of substances in an attempt to overcome this problem. Addition of glycine, or a combination of calcium carbonate and citric acid, aids disintegration of the tablet and improve solubility. A popular effervescent preparation contains citric acid and an excess of sodium bicarbonate. The only two preparations which appear to reduce the incidence of gastric bleeding are enteric-coated tablets and polymerized aluminium aspirin (aloxiprin), but the former may appear unchanged in the stools. Up to 70 per cent of healthy subjects have occult blood in the faeces on taking therapeutic doses of aspirin. Dyspepsia occurs in a third of patients given aspirin in full doses for rheumatoid arthritis and makes it no longer the drug of first choice in this disease. Furthermore, chronic occult blood loss may lead to iron deficiency anaemia. Occasionally dramatic haemorrhage occurs from acute gastric erosion. A considerable proportion of patients admitted to hospital with haematemesis give a history of recent ingestion of aspirin or another mild analgesic.

Aspirin is a powerful anti-inflammatory drug, having antihistamine, anti-5HT and antikinin properties. It also inhibits the synthesis of prostaglandins (p. 138). It is antipyretic, probably acting directly on the hypothalamus, but despite this it increases the metabolic rate, and on overdosage can cause hyperpyrexia. It has a variety of metabolic effects, inhibiting enzymes in Krebs cycle and producing hypoglycaemia or hyperglycaemia, glycosuria and ketosis on overdosage. Salicysm, including deafness, tinnitus, nausea and dizziness, occurs with high doses.

Acute poisoning causes vomiting, headache, hyperpyrexia, hyperventilation, flushing of the skin and sweating. Large doses cause acidaemia and hypokalaemia, which probably account for the occurrence of pulmonary oedema, cardiovascular collapse and sudden death coma is unusual. Aspirin poisoning accounts for 15 per cent of all cases of overdosage. Mortality is higher in children than in adults. Other toxic effects include toxic amblyopia, and haemorrhage reversed by vitamin K. Allergic reactions to aspirin are not uncommon and include bronchial asthma, urticaria and vasomotor rhinitis.

Diflunisal is a fluorinated salicylate with a longer analgesic action than aspirin, permitting twice daily administration. It appears to cause less gastrointestinal adverse effects than aspirin, but gastric haemorrhage has been described, and it can potentiate the action of warfarin and similar anticoagulants.

Salsalate is hydrolysed after absorption to salicylic acid, and has similar properties to aspirin. Sodium salicylate is also available for oral administration.

Methylsalicylate is a highly irritant substance, suitable only for application to the skin as a rubefacient.

Paracetamol (Acetaminophen)
The analgesic effect of this drug is slightly less than that of aspirin. It does not produce gastric irritation, nor does it cause haemolytic anaemia or methaemoglobinaemia as does phenacetin. It is a relatively safe drug, but liver damage can occur with acute poisoning with more than 15 g of the drug (p. 256). It has negligible anti-inflammatory properties. Benorylate is a chemical combination of aspirin and paracetamol which is claimed to circumvent the gastric irritant properties of the former constituent. Enzymatic cleavage in the liver breaks the chemical link.

Anthranilic acid derivatives
These include mefenamic acid and flufenamic acid. They have a minor anti-inflammatory effect and are therefore satisfactory for symptomic relief in the early stages of rheumatoid arthritis, but their range of effect is very limited. Gastro-intestinal effects, particularly diarrhoea, are common.

Proprionic acid derivatives
Ibuprofen, ketoprofen, fenoprofen, benoxaprofen, naproxen and

flurbiprofen are weak to moderate anti-inflammatory drugs which are valuable in mild rheumatoid arthritis. Naproxen is particularly effective and its low incidence of adverse effects makes it a drug of first choice in the early stages.

Arylacetic acid derivatives
Fenclofenac, alclofenac and diclofenac possess weak to moderate anti-inflammatory activity and possess a similar spectrum of activity to the propronic acid derivatives.

Indomethacin
Indomethacin is a major anti-inflammatory drug which is widely used in musculo-skeletal and inflammatory joint conditions. It can be used in high doses for short periods of time, e.g. in the treatment of an acute exacerbation of gout; in a single large dose last thing at night to prevent early morning stiffness in rheumatoid arthritis; or daily in divided maintenance doses for inflammatory disorders. When used in the latter way, adverse effects are relatively common, including headache, vertigo, depression and mental confusion. Gastro-intestinal disturbances include anorexia, abdominal pain and peptic ulceration with perforation or haemorrhage. Sulindac is a related drug but with a milder effect. Tolmetin is a pyrrole acetic acid derivative with a similar spectrum of activity to indomethacin.

Pyrazolone derivitives
Phenylbutazone and its derivative oxyphenbutazone are potent anti-inflammatory drugs with uricosuric activity, of particular value in the treatment of inflammatory joint conditions including gout. Their use is limited, however, by the high incidence of side-effects which they produce, including nausea and vomiting, skin rashes, peptic ulceration with haemorrhage and perforation, and sodium retention with oedema and hypertension. Their most serious adverse effects are on the bone marrow with thrombocytopenia, agranulocytosis and aplastic anaemia, which occurs in about one in 80 000 administrations. The frequency of these toxic effects appears to be related to the dose administered and it is therefore wise to limit this to not more than 300 mg daily.

Like aspirin, phenylbutazone binds strongly to plasma proteins and may potentiate the actions of other drugs such as the oral anticoagulants by displacement.

Azapropazone and feprazone are chemically related to phenylbutazone but have a milder anti-inflammatory effect resembling the proprionic acid derivatives. They do not produce blood dyscrasias.

Choice of mild analgesic

Newer preparations have not displaced aspirin from its position as the safest and cheapest of mild analgesics for headaches and musculo-skeletal pains. Some patients, however, are intolerant of it either because of dyspepsia or, less commonly, a hypersensitivity reaction. For these patients paracetamol is a satisfactory substitute except in inflammatory conditions, where its value is limited to simple analgesia. Codeine is often as effective, or more so, than aspirin, but it is unsatisfactory for continuous use as it produces constipation. A number of preparations combine aspirin, paracetamol, codeine or dextropropoxyphene. Although as a general rule it is better to use a single drug rather than mixtures, these preparations are satisfactory even though the effects of the analgesics are simply additive. Preparations which combine mild analgesics and tranquillizers, sedatives, stimulants or muscle relaxants should be avoided.

Dihydrocodeine is more powerful than aspirin but, like codeine, it produces constipation, and it makes some patients dizzy and sleepy.

Choice of anti-inflammatory analgesic

In the early stages of rheumatoid arthritis, simple mild analgesic therapy is all that is required. Aspirin in low doses is usually well tolerated, but in full anti-inflammatory doses gastrointestinal upsets are common. A satisfactory first choice in mild disease is a proprionic acid derivative such as naproxen, but in more advanced disease a drug with a more powerful anti-inflammatory effect is necessary, such as indomethacin or phenylbutazone. If these are ineffective, one of the compounds discussed below may be necessary. Steroid therapy should be a last resort because the adverse effects resulting from long term therapy are so troublesome.

Gout

Gout is a metabolic disorder caused by an inborn error of uric acid metabolism, which produces attacks of painful arthritis and, in advanced stages, deposition of urate crystals in joints, subcutaneous tissues, kidneys and heart.

Treatment of the acute attack

Indomethacin or phenylbutazone are drugs of choice in the treatment of an acute attack, given two hourly until the pain begins to subside. Colchicine, the classical treatment for the acute attack, is used only in patients who are unable to tolerate anti-inflammatory drugs.

Prophylactic treatment

(a) Allopurinol. The formation of uric acid from xanthine and hypoxanthine is catalyzed by the enzyme xanthine oxidase. Allopurinol which resembles hypoxanthine structurally inhibits this enzyme and so reduces uric acid formation and the serum uric acid level falls. Urate deposits may also be reduced. Allopurinol is effective not only in primary gout but also in other conditions in which there is excessive production of uric acid such as polycythaemia and the leukaemias.

(b) Probenecid is a uricosuric drug which acts by inhibiting the renal tubular transport of organic acids. Normally a large proportion of uric acid filtered by the glomerulus is reabsorbed by the renal tubule, and inhibition of this process results in a marked increase in uric acid excretion. This leads to a fall in serum uric acid levels and reduction in urate deposits throughout the body. Probenecid also blocks the secretion of penicillin into the renal tubule, leading to a reduction in penicillin excretion and augmentation of penicillin blood levels after a given dose. Sulphinpyrazone, like probenecid, is a potent inhibitor of renal tubular reabsorption of uric acid. It is now so well tolerated as probenecid, producing gastrointestinal irritation in many patients. Allopurinol has largely replaced uricosuric agents for prophylactic treatment of gout.

Analgesic nephropathy

In some communities abuse of analgesic mixtures containing aspirin, phenacetin or phenazone, and caffeine has developed, largely because of the stimulating property of the latter drug. No true addiction occurs, but considerable psychological dependence can develop. Several grams of these drugs have been consumed daily for many years by devotees of this practice, and this has led in some to characteristic necrotic changes in the renal papillae. This has been labelled 'phenacetin nephritis', but the identity of the drug responsible for this lesion is still disputed. The reason for this is that mixtures of drugs, rather than a single analgesic, have almost invariably been taken, and aspirin or another anti-inflammatory drugs has always been one of the combination. Furthermore, experimental renal lesions in animals have been produced by many mild analgesics, but only with difficulty with phenacetin.

To complicate the picture further, paracetamol has recently been incriminated. It may be that all these drugs contribute, but whatever the truth it will be some time before this problem is resolved. In the meantime, patients should be discouraged from chronic ingestion of any mild analgesic, whether alone or contained in a mixture.

Carcinoma of the renal papillae has been reported in patients who have abused these drugs, and this may be related to chronic irritation of the papillary epithelium.

Other drugs used in rheumatoid arthritis

Gold salts

Gold salts appear to be of value in the treatment of some patients with active rheumatoid arthritis, but are not effective in other joint diseases. The most commonly used is gold sodium thiomalate (sodium aurothiomalate, Myocrisin), a suspension in oil given by intramuscular injection in prolonged courses. Large amounts are retained in the body particularly in the liver, spleen and kidneys, and excretion is chiefly in the urine. Gold may be detected in the urine for as long as 15 months after a course of treatment. Toxic reactions are common, the most frequent being stomatitis and dermatitis. Nausea, vomiting and diarrhoea are also relatively frequent. More serious toxic effects include hepatitis, nephritis and bone marrow depression with thrombocytopenia, agranulocytosis and aplastic anaemia. Gold salts should not be given to patients with a history of kidney or liver dysfunction.

Antimalarial drugs

Some antimalarial drugs also possess therapeutic anti-inflammatory activity, the most commonly used being chloroquine and hydroxychloroquine. Their chief indications for this purpose are rheumatoid arthritis and discoid or systematic lupus erythematosis. They have also been used in sarcoidosis but with questionable results. Long-term administration is required in these conditions, and may result in adverse effects including exfoliative skin reactions with increased pigmentation, alopecia and bleaching of the hair, and peripheral neuropathy. The most serious adverse effects of chronic treatment are on the eye, with development of corneal opacities and pigmentary disturbances in the macula associated with loss of central visual acuity and blindness which is irreversible. Because of these serious effects, their use is restricted to severe disease.

D-*Penicillamine*

This compound is used to chelate copper in Wilson's disease, but a favourable response has been found in patients with rheumatoid arthritis. Its effect may be related to reduction in sulphydryl groups. It is usually reserved for patients who have responded poorly to more conventional therapy and who have troublesome extra-articular features such as vasculitis. Toxic effects are common, and include rashes, purpura, thrombocytopenia, leucopenia, proteinuria associated with immune complex nephritis and loss of taste.

Immunostimulant drugs

Levamisole is an immunostimulant drug which is undergoing evaluation in rheumatoid arthritis.

Immunosuppressive drugs

Immunosuppressive and cytoxic drugs such as azathioprine, chlorambucil and methotrexate are used in some progressive and potentially fatal inflammatory conditions in which it is believed that an autoimmune mechanism is at work—such as systemic lupus erythematosis and the nephrotic syndrome—when other treatment failed to produce a therapeutic response. They can be used as alternatives in cases of rheumatoid arthritis that have failed to respond to gold and penicillamine. It is not yet certain, however, whether any therapeutic effect that is seen is, in fact, due to suppression of immune mechanisms rather than a non-specific anti-inflammatory effect of the drugs used.

Corticosteroids

Steroid hormones secreted by the adrenal cortex may be subdivided into (a) glucocorticoids, such as hydrocortisone and cortisone which exert their chief effect on fat, protein and carbohydrate metabolism and possess marked anti-inflammatory activity, and (b) mineralocorticoids, such as desoxycorticosterone and aldosterone, which are concerned primarily with electrolyte and water balance. In addition to their glucocorticoid effects, hydrocortisone and cortisone both have marked mineralocorticoid actions, which are a disadvantage when they are being used as anti-inflammatory agents. Newer synthetic steroids have much less.

Cortisone was originally isolated from adrenal extracts but is now synthesized for therapeutic use. It is rapidly hydroxylated to hydrocortisone (cortisol) by the liver, and is used only for replacement therapy in Addison's disease. Hydrocortisone is believed to be the most important naturally secreted glucocorticoid hormone of the adrenal cortex. Prednisolone, prednisone (which is hydroxylated to prednisolone after absorption), triamcinolone, dexamethasone and betamethasone possess greater anti-inflammatory properties without an increase in salt retaining activity (see Table 15).

Corticosteroids demonstrate the following actions:

(a) Atrophy of the adrenal cortex, with the exception of the zona glomerulosa, and depression of normal adrenal cortical function. This is due to suppression of release of adrenocorticotrophic hormone from the pituitary gland, due in turn to suppression of corticotrophin-releasing factor from the hypothalamus.

(b) Retention of sodium and increased loss of potassium from the body. Adrenal cortical insufficiency is associated with sodium loss, hyponatraemia, hyperkalaemia, and a reduction in the extracellular fluid volume. These changes are reversed by adrenal steroid hormones, particularly the mineralacorticoids such as aldosterone. In the normal subject sodium retention leads to increased body weight, hypertension and oedema.

Table 15

	Relative anti-inflammatory activity (glucocorticoid)	Relative salt-retaining potency (mineralocorticoid)
Cortisone	1	1
Hydrocortisone	1	1
Prednisone	5	1
Prednisolone	5	1
Triamcinolone	5	<1
Dexamethasone	35	<1
Betamethasone	35	<1

(c) Increased gluconeogenesis through mobilization of protein and amino acids from skeletal muscle.

(d) Shrinkage of lymphoid tissue and reduction in lymphocyte production leading to a lymphocytopenia in the blood.

(e) Reduction in the blood eosinophil count and rise in the neutrophil granulocyte count.

(f) Suppression of the inflammatory response.

The *clinical indications* for systemic treatment with corticosteroids are:

1. Replacement therapy in patients with adrenal cortical insufficiency due to Addison's disease, the Waterhouse-Friderichsen syndrome or post-adrenalectomy. It is usual to combine treatment

with a synthetic mineralocorticoid compound such as fludrocortisone with cortisone. The salt retaining activity of prednisolone or one of the other synthetic glucocorticoids is not sufficient for satisfactory replacement therapy.

2. Treatment with pharmacological doses of steroids.

(i) Shrinkage of lymphatic tissue and suppression of lymphopoiesis in patients with leukaemias and lymphomas.

(ii) Suppression of the rejection phenomenon in tissue transplantation.

(iii) Anti-inflammatory therapy in a variety of conditions including rheumatoid arthritis, systemic lupus erythematosis, polyarteritis, dermatomyositis, ulcerative colitis, sarcoidosis, the nephrotic syndrome, bronchial asthma (see p. 154), severe inflammatory conditions of the eye and skin, cerebral oedema and raised intracranial pressure. Corticosteroids are also used in the treatment of autoimmune haemolytic anaemia and thrombocytopenic purpura.

For replacement therapy cortisone, hydrocortisone and fludrocortisone are the preparations of choice. For the treatment of leukaemia, lymphoma and inflammatory conditions steroids with more potent effects but with relatively less salt retaining properties are used, particularly prednisolone or prednisone. As prednisone is converted to prednisolone after absorption, it is rational to regard prednisolone as the standard drug of choice for these indications. It may be administered orally, intravenously, by enema, intra-articularly, or locally to the eye and skin. The more potent steroids dexamethasone and betamethasone are used where very high doses are required to suppress the inflammatory reaction or other disease process, and in local conditions of the eye and skin. Dexamethasone is used to suppress the adrenal cortex in tests of pituitary–adrenal function and to reduce raised intracranial pressure caused by brain oedema associated with, for example, brain tumour or status epilepticus.

Adverse effects of corticosteroid therapy

The following complications of corticosteroid therapy may be seen, particularly in the high doses required for anti-inflammatory activity. They are not seen in replacement doses for adrenocortical insufficiency.

1. Fulminating infections. The normal inflammatory responses to bacterial and viral infection are reduced or masked. Latent tuberculous foci may be reactivated.

2. Osteoporosis and collapse of vertebrae due to mobilization of tissue proteins in gluconeogenesis.

3. Myopathy with muscle weakness and wasting, especially involving the proximal girdle muscles. This is especially prominent with triamcinolone.

4. Diabetes mellitus due to gluconeogenesis and increased insulin resistance.

5. Hypertension, due to sodium and water retention. This may proceed to cardiac failure.

6. Weight gain, oedema, bruising, purple striae in the skin particularly of the abdomen, moon face.

7. Psychotic reactions of all types may occur.

8. Hirsutism and menstrual disturbances.

9. Pancreatitis.

10. Cataracts may be seen after long-term treatment.

11. Retardation of growth may be seen after long term use in children.

12. Withdrawal phenomena. The adrenal suppression accompanying steroid therapy leads to symptoms and signs of adrenal insufficiency if the steroid is abruptly withdrawn. These are anorexia, nausea, vomiting, diarrhoea, abdominal pain, headache, arthralgia, restlessness, lethargy, muscle weakness, temperature disturbances, dehydration, hypotension and vascular collapse. The condition is treated with saline infusion and administration or fludrocortisone and hydrocortisone.

Therapeutic use of corticosteroids has been thought to cause peptic ulceration, although this is questionable.

Interactions involving corticosteroids–see page 29.

Corticotrophins

Corticotrophin (adrenocorticotrophic hormone) is a polypeptide secreted by the anterior pituitary gland under the influence of corticotrophin-releasing factor from the hypothalamus. It stimulates the adrenal cortex to secrete hydrocortisone and other hormones, and is administered parenterally by intramuscular or intravenous injection as its activity is rapidly destroyed by proteolytic enzymes in the gastrointestinal tract. Long-acting preparations of corticotrophin in gelatin solution or adsorbed on to zinc hydroxide are available for daily intramuscular injection.

Synthetic corticotrophic hormones which consist of part of the peptide chain of natural corticotrophin have been prepared, for example, tetracosactrin. They are preferable for use in patients who show hypersensitivity to natural corticotrophin, although hypersensitivity reactions to the synthetic agent have been described, albeit rarely. There is evidence that it may be absorbed through the nasal mucosa when administered as snuff.

Corticotrophins may be used in those conditions for which corticosteroids are given, apart from adrenal cortical replacement therapy. Such treatment involves regular injections, however, which is less convenient particularly in long-term therapy, and most physicians prefer to use oral corticosteroids. In children corticotrophin may be preferable because there is evidence that it retards growth less than corticosteroids. Adrenal suppression does not follow the use of corticotrophin as it does with corticosteroids, and patients treated with it tend to retain a normal adrenal response to stress. Hypertension, pigmentation, hirsutism and acne occur more frequently as complications of corticotrophin therapy because it stimulates the production of androgenic steroids as well as cortisol. Dyspepsia, bruising, striae formation, osteoporosis and myopathy are less frequent with corticotrophin.

ANTIHISTAMINES

Histamine receptors can be subdivided into H_1 - and H_2-receptors. The latter are found in the stomach and atria, and are not blocked by the traditional antihistamine drugs. Some newer compounds appear to be selective on H_2-receptors and are receiving clinical trials in the treatment of gastric ulcer. The account which follows is confined to the traditional antihistamines. H_2-receptor antagonists are discussed in Chapter 12.

The number of proprietary antihistamine preparations is enormous, but, as is usual in these circumstances, there are only minor differences between them. It is an easy matter to produce a useful antihistamine, which is the reason why most drug companies market at least one. Antihistamine properties are ubiquitous among compounds belonging to other pharmacological groups, including phenothiazine tranquillizers, antidepressants and α-adrenergic blocking drugs. Likewise, antihistamines have many other pharmacological actions (Table 16). Briefly their pharmacology can be summarized as follows:

(a) Antihistamine effect. This is a competitive antagonism, and must be contrasted with the physiological reversal of histamine actions by adrenaline. Although the bronchoconstrictor and vasodilator effects of histamine are antagonized, the histamine-induced

Table 16

	Sedative effect	Anticholinergic effect	Anti-metic effect	Other uses
Promethazine	+++	+++	++	Sedative, hypnotic, anti-emetic
Diphenhydramine	+++	+++	++	
Cyproheptadine	++	++	Minimal	Appetite stimulant, 5HT antagonist
Cyclizine	+	+	+++	Anti-emetic
Meclozine	+	+	+++	Anti-emetic
Mepyramine	+	+	o	
Chlorpheniramine	+	++	Minimal	
Phenindamine	Minimal	++	Minimal	
Clemastine	Minimal	+	Not evaluated	

gastric acid production, mediated through H_2 receptors, is not inhibited (see p. 159).

(b) Anticholinergic properties. These produce peripheral atropine-like adverse effects, such as dryness of the mouth, blurred vision and tachycardia. They may account also for the value of some antihistamines as anti-emetic and anti-Parkinsonian drugs, although two of the most powerful anti-emetics, meclozine and cyclizine, have weak peripheral atropine-like effects. Diphenhydramine and phenindamine have been used in Parkinsonism, but their effects are mild compared with those of other anticholinergics. Antihistamines with marked anticholinergic actions, such as diphenhydramine and promethazine, should not be given to patients with glaucoma or prostatic hypertrophy.

(c) α-Adrenergic and 5HT blocking actions are possessed particularly by the phenothiazine derivative promethazine. Cyproheptadine, related structurally to imipramine, has potent anti-5HT effects, and has been used to antagonize the peripheral effects of 5HT secreted by carcinoid tumours. It stimulates appetite.

(d) Local anaesthetic actions. This is most marked with antazoline, which has been used as an antidysrhythmic.

(e) Central effects. Sedation is one of the main drawbacks of most antihistamines, and the major effort in the development of these compounds has been concentrated on producing a non-sedative drug. Promethazine and diphenhydramine are the worst from this point of view, although this is of value when the former drug is used as a long acting hypnotic. Phenindamine, clemastine, chlorpheniramine and terfenadine are generally considered to be better in this respect than most antihistamines. Patients should be advised to avoid alcohol and other central depressant drugs, whose actions are increased by antihistamines, and drivers should be warned of these effects. Despite their sedative properties some antihistamines have convulsant properties and should not, if possible, be used in epileptics.

(f) Other actions. Topical use of these drugs can cause photosensitivity and other skin eruptions, and should be avoided. Gastrointestinal disturbances occur occasionally, including epigastric distress, anorexia, nausea and constipation or diarrhoea. Agranulocytosis, haemolytic anaemia and thrombocytopenia occur rarely. Cyclizine and meclozine are under suspicion as possible teratogenic agents, and should therefore be avoided in women of child-bearing age.

Indications for use

Antihistamines are of most value when histamine plays a major role in the clinical syndrome produced by an immune reaction. This is the case in acute allergic responses to drugs, chemicals, certain foodstuffs and pollen, producing acute urticarial reactions and seasonal hay-fever. These conditions are considerably relieved by oral administration of an antihistamine and withdrawal, if possible, of the allergen. A generalized anaphylactic reaction requires more urgent action, and here administration of subcutaneous adrenaline is essential. Antihistamines are only of supplementary benefit, partly because other substances, e.g. various kinins, may be involved in this reaction. Similarly, angioneurotic oedema is better treated with adrenaline, for although it is improved by antihistamines they do not act quickly enough in a life-threatening situation.

Pruritus is relieved only when it is caused by histamine release, as in the itching accompanying acute urticaria, and following insect bites. If the lesions are localized, application of antihistamine ointment are of great value, but repeated and extensive use should be discouraged because of the risk of photosensitivity. Pruritus not caused by histamine release is better treated by a phenothiazine.

Chronic urticaria and chronic allergies, e.g. contact dermatitis, are less often helped. Similarly, antihistamines are of little value in serum sickness, although accompanying urticarial skin lesions may be improved.

Bronchial asthma does not respond to oral or intravenous antihistamines, even when there is an obvious allergic cause such as pollen sensitivity. The only exception to this is bronchospasm from the release of histamine by drugs, such as dextran and tubocurarine, although even in this case adrenaline is more effective. The course of a common cold is not influenced by antihistamines, although their atropine-like effects may reduce nasal secretions to some extent.

The use of antihistamines as anti-emetics is discussed on page 86.

Choice of drug

The main consideration in choosing an antihistamine is whether or not sedation is desirable. Occasionally it is, as for instance in an acute urticarial reaction or in a patient who is being kept awake by itching. But in most cases it is undesirable, e.g. in a patient who continues to work or drive while receiving an antihistamine for hay-fever. There is considerable variation in response to the various antihistamines. One patient may be sedated by one drug, whereas another patient is not. It is therefore worthwhile trying several drugs in patients who will need prolonged administration.

17

Vitamins and iron

Vitamins are essential constituents of the diet because, excepting vitamin D and nicotinic acid, they cannot be synthesized in the body. Vitamins B and C are water soluble, whereas vitamins A, D and K are fat soluble and likely to be malabsorbed in steatorrhoea. Although the consumption of vitamin preparations is enormous, the clinical indications for their administration are few.

Vitamin A

Dietary vitamin A comes from animal sources, particularly liver and dairy produce, and from certain vegetables such as carrots and tomatoes. Margarine is reinforced with vitamins A and D. The daily requirement is about 2500 iu, with a higher intake during pregnancy and lactation. In Britain deficiency of this vitamin is rare, and is almost always associated with malabsorption and steatorrhea, but in some underdeveloped countries it is common.

Vitamin A has two essential functions, (a) it is a constituent part of visual purple (rhodopsin); and (b) it plays an important part in the maintenance of epithelial surfaces. Severe deficiency of the vitamin can cause a defect in dark adaptation, leading to night blindness, and conversion of mucous surfaces into stratified squamous epithelium. When the cornea and conjunctiva are involved xerophthalmia and keratomalacia can occur if the condition remains untreated.

For treatment of deficiency disease 50 000 iu should be administered daily until the symptoms have resolved. Prophylactic vitamin A, usually in conjunction with vitamin D, is often given to pregnant and lactating women, and to infants. Chronic ingestion of large quantities of the vitamin can produce toxicity, manifested by irritability, loss of appetite, itching and hypoprothrombinaemia. Peeling of the skin can occur in acute intoxication, as occurred in Arctic explorers who ate polar bear liver.

Vitamin B group

Four vitamins of this group will be dealt with together because a deficiency of one is usually accompanied by a deficiency of the others, and clinical syndromes are often mixed. These include thiamine hydrochloride (aneurine, B_1), riboflavine (B_2), pyridoxine (B_6) and nicotinic acid (B_7). Folic acid and cyanocobalamin (B_{12}) are dealt with separately below.

Thiamine is of importance as a coenzyme in the decarboxylation of pyruvic acid. The clinical deficiency syndrome includes cardiac failure (wet beri-beri), peripheral neuritis (dry beri-beri) and Wernicke's encephalopathy (cerebral beri-beri). It is a disease of under-developed countries, but is occasionally seen in Britain, particularly in alcoholics. Cardiac beri-beri usually responds dramatically to administration of physiological amounts of thiamine, and the diagnosis is probably often overlooked, for a normal ward diet contains sufficient of the B vitamins to overcome the deficiency in a few days. Neurological forms of the disease respond more slowly, especially the peripheral neuritis, probably because factors other than thiamine deficiency are involved.

Riboflavine acts as a coenzyme for a variety of respiratory enzymes. Its deficiency leads to angular stomatitis and ulceration of mucous membranes, but is usually accompanied by other B vitamin deficiency diseases. In Britain angular stomatitis is usually caused by factors other than riboflavine deficiency.

Pyridoxine is converted to pyridoxal phosphate in the body and acts as a coenzyme to transaminases. Pyridoxine deficiency can cause fits in infancy. Rarely, familial pyridoxine resistance occurs. Large doses of pyridoxine are sometimes of value in sideroblastic anaemia, which is a type of hypochromic anaemia in which the adequate stores of iron in the bone marrow cannot be incorporated into red cells.

Nicotinic acid is an essential component of co-dehydrogenases I and II. Deficiency of this vitamin causes pellagra, with its classical trio of symptoms, dermatitis, dementia and diarrhoea. It is extremely rare in Britain, although it is occasionally seen in patients with disturbed tryptophan metabolism (e.g. during isoniazid therapy) for nicotinic acid is normally synthesized endogenously from tryptophan as well as being absorbed from the diet. Nicotinic acid can cause flushing of the blush areas when used in large doses to treat hypercholesterolaemia.

Indications for use
The use of these four vitamins, either alone, or in a multi-vitamin preparation is indicated only in a few well defined circumstances.

(a) *Dietary deficiency*. The average diet of the British population contains generous amounts of these vitamins and therefore the use of tonics and other preparations containing them is entirely unnecessary in a healthy person receiving a normal diet. Intake can become critical or frankly inadequate in two types of person, the alcoholic and the elderly person living alone. Obviously the best treatment is to ensure an adequate diet, but the use of vitamin supplements has a place, particularly in the immediate treatment of a clinical deficiency. For this purpose a parenteral multivitamin preparation (Parenterovite) is generally used.

(b) *Malabsorption*. Deficiency of the B vitamins is unusual in malabsorption, but supplements are occasionally necessary when treatment fails to control the malabsorptive state.

(c) *Prolonged vomiting and intravenous feeding*. Parenteral treatment with B vitamins may be necessary in hyperemesis gravidarum, gastrointestinal disease or following major surgery.

(d) *Antibiotic treatment*. Isoniazid can interfere with the metabolism of pyridoxine and can cause peripheral neuritis when prolonged courses are given, as is usual when the drug is used for treating tuberculosis. It occurs only when the serum level of the drug is excessive, as in slow acetylators. Prophylactic pyridoxine may be necessary when higher doses of isoniazid are given. The adverse effects of tetracline administration, such as sore mouth and diarrhoea, are not the result of vitamin deficiency.

Folic acid

In contrast to the other vitamins of the B group, deficiency of folic acid is relatively common. Although severe deficiency can cause megaloblastic anaemia, there is some evidence that a milder deficiency can produce more general symptoms such as malaise and anorexia, but no adequately controlled studies have been performed. There may also be a connection between folate deficiency and certain obstetric complications and foetal abnormalities.

Serum and red cell levels of folate can be readily measured with microbiological assays. The red cell level is more representative of the tissue stores of folate than the serum level, which fluctuates with dietary intake. The daily requirement of an adult is about 50–75 μg, and the average diet contains two or three times this amount. In the last trimester of pregnancy, however, the physiological requirement is increased to 150–200 μg/day and therefore a deficiency can easily occur when the diet is below standard. Mild folate deficiency is so common in pregnancy that it is standard practice in most obstetric units to prescribe a folic acid supplement.

Other causes of folate deficiency are malabsorption, certain diseases in which folate requirements are increased, such as malignancy, leukaemias, chronic inflammatory conditions and psoriasis, and certain substances which interfere with folate metabolism, such as anticonvulsant drugs, nitrofurantoin and folic acid antagonists.

Indications for use

There are two indications for administration of folic acid, (a) to treat established deficiency and (b) as prophylaxis in conditions known to be associated with an increased requirement for the vitamin.

(a) Established deficiency is treated with 5–15 mg of folic acid (pteroylmonoglutamic acid) daily to replete body stores. The subsequent maintenance dose depends upon the body requirement. This seldom exceeds 300 ug/day, but in practice much larger doses are given. Up to 50 per cent of patients on anticonvulsant drugs have low folate levels, but megaloblastic anaemia is rare. There is little evidence that replacement therapy helps in any way in the absence of megaloblastic anaemia.

Folic acid should never be given alone when the serum level of vitamin B_{12} is low, as in Addisonian pernicious anaemia, because neurological complications can be precipitated despite haematological improvement. Physiological doses (100 ug) of folic acid are often used as a therapeutic trial to confirm the cause of a patient's megaloblastic anaemia.

(b) Prophylaxis in pregnancy is justified by the frequency with which haematological evidence of anaemia occurs, and by the possible role of folate deficiency in causing obstetric complications. It is usual to give a combined iron and folic acid preparation, although the optimum dose of each is a matter for dispute. Proprietary preparations contain from 100 ug to 5 mg of folic acid and 30 to 150 mg of iron.

Treatment with cytostatic folic acid antagonists may produce signs of folate deficiency for which folinic acid may be required.

Vitamin B_{12}

The average daily intake of vitamin B_{12} is 5–10 ug and this is greatly in excess of the body requirement. Dietary deficiency is therefore rare. Clinical deficiency disease is seen when there is malabsorption due to lack of intrinsic factor (pernicious anaemia), following total or partial gastrectomy, or in various small bowel diseases. The effects of vitamin B_{12} deficiency are megaloblastic anaemia, peripheral neuropathy and subacute combined degeneration of the spinal cord, and dementia. Administration of the vitamin is indicated in several circumstances.

(a) Established deficiency, of whatever cause, should be treated with several injections of 1000 μg at intervals of a few days between each injection in order to replete the liver stores of the vitamin. Maintenance doses of 250 μg/month are more than adequate to meet the daily requirement. In megaloblastic anaemia caused by vitamin B_{12} deficiency a brisk reticulocyte response is seen, reaching a peak at about 7 days after the start of treatment. A single dose as small as 100 ng is enough to produce a reticulocyte response, and this can be a useful diagnostic test. Improvement of neurological lesions is slow and often incomplete.

(b) Prophylaxis is given in patients who will, or might, become deficient as a result of gastric surgery. This is an inevitable result of total gastrectomy.

(c) Leber's optic atrophy and tobacco amblyopia respond to large doses of vitamin B_{12}.

Vitamin B_{12} is available as cyanocobalamin or hydroxocobalamin. The latter is the more satisfactory preparation as it is retained in the body more readily.

Vitamin C (ascorbic acid)

The main function of this vitamin is the conversion of proline to hydroxyproline, which is an important constituent of collagen and intercellular substance. When it is lacking intercellular substance becomes thin and watery, giving little support to blood vessels in tissues, and as a result petichial haemorrhages and ecchymoses occur. The gums become inflamed and swollen. Lack of collagen in bone causes easy fracturing and poor healing. Anaemia, of either a macrocytic or normocytic type, can occur. This clinical syndrome is called scurvy.

The daily requirement is 20–30 mg/day, but scurvy does not occur unless the daily intake is below 10 mg for many months. Deficiency is rare, and is confined to the elderly and the very young. The vitamin is found exclusively in fruit and vegetables, the potato being the main dietary source. Many fruit drinks are supplemented with vitamin C. A high intake results in a high urinary excretion.

Indication for use

Administration of vitamin C is necessary only when deficiency has been diagnosed or, prophylactically, when the diet is deficient in the vitamin, e.g. in infants and the elderly. Patients with a subclinical deficiency show delayed healing of wounds after surgery, and for this reason some surgeons prescribe the vitamin routinely. It is often used in the common cold and other infections, although the evidence that it promotes recovery is equivocal.

Vitamin D

Included under this name are several steroid compounds which have antirachitic properties. Vitamin D_2 (ergocalciferol) is derived by ultraviolet irradiation of a provitamin (ergosterol) of vegetable origin and is the most widely used clinically. Dihydrotachysterol is derived from the same provitamin. Vitamin D_3 (cholecalciferol) is produced by irradiation of 7-dehydrocholesterol, a provitamin of animal origin which is found in the Malpighian layer of the human skin, and which is converted to cholecalciferol by sunlight. This vitamin is found also in milk and fish liver oils, and is added to margarine.

The antirachitic activity of these vitamins is dependent upon their conversion into active metabolites by hydroxylation in the liver and kidneys (Fig. 19). 25-Hydroxycholecalciferol is produced

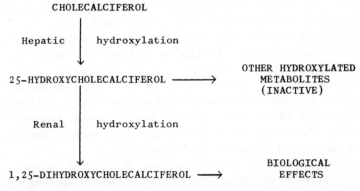

Fig. 19 Activation of cholecalciferol (vitamin D_3) in liver and kidneys.

in the liver, and this is further hydroxylated to 1,25-dihydroxy-cholecalciferol by the kidneys. These are the chief active metabolites. Other more polar metabolites are produced, but are biologically inactive. Anticonvulsant drugs interfere with hepatic hydroxylation, leading to accelerated production of inactive metabolites. Renal disease can impair the production of the dihydroxy derivative. In both these situations osteomalacia can occur.

Rickets in childhood results from an inadequate dietary intake and lack of exposure to sunlight, and was common in the industrial cities of Victorian England. Familial vitamin D resistance is occasionally seen. In adults, deficiency can result from disease of the biliary tract or intestine, for vitamin D is fat soluble and will be lost when steatorrhoea exists.

Vitamin D promotes the intestinal absorption of calcium and phosphorous, their mobilization from bone and possibly their renal excretion. Serum calcium levels are increased, and hypercalcaemia can occur with overdosage, producing renal calcinosis and renal failure. The metabolic effects of vitamin D and parathormone are closely interrelated.

A daily intake of 10 μg (400 iu) is adequate during childhood, pregnancy and lactation. In adults 5 μg is probably adequate, but the average diet contains considerably greater amounts than this. Exposure to sunlight has a potent antirachitic effect.

Indications for use

(a) Treatment of rickets and osteomalacia. Physiological doses will promote rapid healing when the diet has been deficient. In practice up to 250 μg daily are given, but it is important to avoid too high a dose. Renal calcinosis can occur with chronic intake of 1 mg daily. When bone disease has been caused by bowel disease, renal disease or familial vitamin D resistance much larger doses may be required, up to 10 mg daily. Frequent estimation of the serum calcium level is necessary. 1α-Hydroxycholecalciferol (alfacalcidol) has been synthesized and appears to be particularly useful in osteomalacia due to renal disease, in which the 1-hydroxylase mechanism is impaired. It has a rapid onset of effect and is useful in the early management of patients with symptoms of hypocalcaemia. Overdosage can occur with prolonged use, but stopping treatment soon reverses the metabolic changes.

(b) Treatment of hypoparathyroidism. Parathyroid hormone is extracted from parathyroid glands but is too antigenic for long term use (see p. 186). Large doses (1–5 mg) of vitamin D are used, often with calcium supplements, to maintain the serum calcium level. Regular monitoring of plasma calcium is necessary to avoid intoxication.

(c) Prophylaxis in infants and pregnant or lactating women is usually recommended, although a normal diet contains an adequate amount of the vitamin. The children of coloured immigrants in Britain occasionally develop rickets, and it is assumed that the skin pigmentation of these patients prevents the compensatory effect of ultraviolet irradiation of the skin.

Vitamin K

Vitamin K is responsible for the production of prothrombin and clotting factors VII, IX and X. It is found in a variety of foods of animal and plant origin, and is synthesized by the normal gut flora. It is available for administration in several forms, the naturally occurring phytomenadione and the synthetic forms menaphthone, menadiol and acetomenaphthone. The synthetic derivatives can cause haemolysis in large doses.

Indications for use

(a) Reversal of anticoagulation. Coumarin and indanedione anticoagulants inhibit the production of prothrombin and factors VII, IX and X. This can be overcome by vitamin K when haemorrhagic complications demand immediate action. Phytomenadione is the most satisfactory for this purpose.

(b) Haemorrhagic disease of the newborn. Low levels of prothrombin and factors VII, IX and X are found in the newborn because of the lack of normal intestinal flora. This is exaggerated in premature infants, and may cause haemorrhagic complications. Routine prophylactic vitamin K is given in many centres. Synthetic analogues displace bilirubin from its plasma-protein binding sites, causing kernicterus if too large a dose is given.

(c) Jaundice. Naturally-occurring vitamin K is fat soluble and requires bile for its normal absorption. Hypoprothrombinaemia accompanying obstructive jaundice responds rapidly to administration of vitamin K, but when liver disease is present the response may be poor.

(d) Intestinal disorders. Hypoprothrombinaemia can occur in steatorrhoea, and when the bacterial flora of the gut are disturbed by oral sulphonamide or broad-spectrum antibiotic treatment.

Iron

The daily requirement of iron is 1 mg in men and 2–3 mg in menstruating women. The absorption from the gut is regulated to the requirement, but although an excess of iron is contained in the average diet much of it is unavailable for absorption. Iron preparations contain ferrous salts which are readily available. Iron deficiency anaemia can occur with a poor diet, with gastrointestinal disorders, during pregnancy or in chronic blood loss. Even a good diet needs supplementing with iron salts in the treatment of established anaemia, for the body stores of about 1500 mg have been depleted.

Oral iron preparations. A number of ferrous salts can be used

Ferrous sulphate is the cheapest, and is satisfactory for most patients. Most preparations contain 50–60 mg of iron. Sometimes it produces nausea, particularly when taken on an empty stomach. In this case ferrous gluconate or fumarate may be tried. Delayed-release preparations reduce gastrointestinal symptoms, but are more expensive and the release of iron from them is less certain. Ferrous succinate is better absorbed than the other salts, and thus the dose is smaller.

Ferric ammonium citrate is available as a liquid preparation, but it can cause blackening of the teeth. Iron edetate is also available, but is expensive.

All iron preparations should be kept out of the reach of children, for they can cause serious acute poisoning.

Interactions with tetracyclines are discussed on p. 25.

Parenteral preparations. Occasionally parenteral preparations are indicated, usually because the patient is considered to be unreliable in drug taking, but sometimes because oral preparations are poorly tolerated or are not absorbed adequately because of gastrointestinal disease. The dose must be calculated from the haemoglobin level, as a large excess can produce haemochromatosis.

Two preparations are available, iron–dextran and iron–sorbitol–citrate. The first of these is the more satisfactory as iron–sorbitol–citrate is partly excreted in the urine. They are given by deep intramuscular injection. A painful local reaction occasionally occurs, and brown staining of the skin is caused by leakage back along the needle track to the subcutaneous tissues. Iron–dextrose can be given as a single replacement dose by intravenous infusion after suitable dilution, although this is seldom required in practice and is associated with a higher incidence of adverse reactions. These include fever, rashes, joint pains, nausea and headache. Anaphylactic shock occurs rarely.

18

Drugs in malignant disease

Alkylating agents

These drugs possess reactive alkyl radicals which link together opposed guanine molecules on the two strands of deoxyribonucleic acid (DNA), preventing the DNA helix uncoiling and so arresting its replication. In this way, mitosis is prevented, particularly in those tissues which show the greatest rate of cell division. In normal subjects this includes the haemopoietic system, the gastrointestinal mucosa and the skin. The faster rate of mitosis in malignant tissues provides the rationale for the use of these drugs in patients with such conditions.

(a) *Mustards.* Mustine hydrochloride, the original nitrogen mustard, was noted to produce leucopenia in subjects dying from exposure to mustard gas in the First World War. It has to be given intravenously, and commonly produces nausea and vomiting within 1 to 4 hours after administration. Pancytopenia occurs with excessive dosage. Its main value is in Hodgkin's disease and lymphosarcoma.

Chlorambucil, a phenylbutyric acid mustard, affects primarily the lymphoid tissues and is of particular value in chronic lymphatic leukaemia, lymphosarcoma and Waldenstrom's macroglobulinaemia. It has also given good results in Hodgkin's disease, ovarian carcinoma and seminoma. Unlike mustine it can be administered orally, and is less damaging to the haemopoietic system, although with excessive dosage or prolonged therapy bone marrow depression may occur.

Melphalan, a phenylalanine mustard, is used mainly in the treatment of myelomatosis.

Cyclophosphamide, a cyclic phosphoramide mustard, is of particular value in Hodgkin's disease, myelomatosis, chronic lymphatic leukaemia and ovarian carcinoma. It produces alopecia more readily than other alkylating agents, and irritant metabolites in the urine may produce a chemical cystitis. It may be given orally or intravenously.

(*b*) *Ethyleneimmonium compounds*. Thiotepa, which is the only important member of this group of alkylating agents, has proved effective in some patients with malignant melanoma, and carcinoma of the breast and ovary. It may be administered orally or intravenously, and may be injected directly into a body cavity containing effusions secondary to metastatic involvement. Like other alkylating agents, prolonged therapy or excessive dosage may produce bone marrow depression.

(*c*) *Dimethanesulphonates*. Busulphan is the most important member of this group and is of particular value in the treatment of chronic myeloid leukaemia, its action in small doses being largely restricted to the myeloid series in the bone marrow, selectively suppressing proliferation of granulocytic cells and to a lesser extent platelet production. It is administered orally, and commonly produces hyperpigmentation of the skin. A rare but important adverse effect is interstitial pulmonary fibrosis similar to that which may follow the use of hexamethonium.

Antimetabolites

An antimetabolite closely resembles a particular metabolite in chemical structure and successfully competes with it as a substrate in an enzyme system. This results in blockade of the particular metabolic pathway involved, which in the case of drugs used in cancer chemotherapy is usually in the synthetic pathway of nucleic acids.

(*a*) *Folic acid antagonists*. Methotrexate competes with folic acid for the enzyme folic acid reductase which is responsible for conversion of folic acid to tetrahydrofolic acid, a coenzyme in the methylation of deoxyuridylic acid to form thymidylic acid. It therefore blocks the synthesis of the latter and consequently of DNA. Its main use is by oral administration in the maintenance treatment of acute lymphoblastic leukaemia, and it may be administered intrathecally to control neurological complications of the disease. It is also very effective in the treatment of chorion carcinoma. When given by intra-arterial perfusion in regional chemotherapy, its systemic toxic effects can be reduced or prevented by parenteral injection of tetrahydrofolic acid. Among its toxic effects are leucopenia and thrombocytopenia, megaloblastic anaemia, alopecia, ulcerative stomatitis and hepatic necrosis and fibrosis.

(*b*) *Purine antagonists*. 6-Mercaptopurine acts at several different points in the early stages of purine synthesis so blocking the production of DNA. Like methotrexate, its most frequent use is in the maintenance treatment of acute leukaemia.

Azathioprine is a derivative of 6-mercaptopurine which is used primarily as an immunosuppressant agent in patients receiving organ transplants.

(c) *Pyrimidine antagonists*. Cytosine arabinoside (cytarabine) interferes with DNA synthesis by blocking the formation of deoxycytidylic acid from cytidylic acid. It is a valuable drug in the treatment of acute myeloblastic leukaemia, particularly when used in combination with other drugs such as daunorubicin. 5-Fluoruracil, like cytarabine, interferes with nucleic acid synthesis and appears to be of benefit in some patients with carcinoma of the ovary, stomach, intestinal tract and breast.

Plant extracts

Colchicine, derived from the autumn crocus, inhibits cell division by arresting mitosis in the metaphase. Although it is not used clinically because of its toxic effects, its derivative demicolcine is sometimes used in chronic myeloid leukaemia and Hodgkin's disease.

Vinca alkaloids come from the West Indian periwinkle. Vinblastine is a valuable drug in the treatment of Hodgkin's disease and chorioncarcinoma, and vincristine is used in combination with prednisolone in the primary treatment of acute lymphoblastic leukaemia. They are administered intravenously. Like colchicine they both cause metaphase arrest. Vincristine is markedly neurotoxic, producing motor, sensory and autonomic neuropathies.

Antibiotics

Actinomycin D, formed during the growth of various *Streptomyces* species, is used in the treatment of Wilm's tumour in children and in chorioncarcinoma and rhabdomyosarcoma. It probably acts by combining with DNA, inhibiting the synthesis of RNA and protein. Daunorubicin (rubidomycin, daunomycin), also derived from certain *Streptomyces* strains, interferes with the synthesis of DNA and RNA by combining with performed DNA. It is one of the most effective drugs in the treatment of acute myeloblastic leukaemia, particularly when used in combination with cytosine arabinoside. It has marked marrow depressant and cardiotoxic properties. Streptozotocin has been successfully used in treating insulin-secreting islet-cell carcinomas of the pancreas. Bleomycin is preferentially concentrated in epithelial tissues and has been used to treat cancers of the mouth and oesophagus, as well as lymphomas. It has been used intrapleurally in patients with mesothelioma of the pleura. It may produce wide-spread lung fibrosis. Cyclosporin A is a potent immunosuppressive agent which is being assessed in transplant surgery to suppress rejection.

Platinum complexes

Platinum diaminodichloride (cis-platinum) appears to inhibit DNA synthesis, and in low concentrations achieves this without significant effect on RNA or protein synthesis. It is given intravenously and distributed throughout all tissues with higher concentrations in liver and kidney. As well as producing nausea, vomiting, bone marrow suppression and immunosuppression, it can also cause renal tubular necrosis and damage to the cochlea. It appears to have a similar spectrum of therapeutic activity to the alkylating agents.

Other drugs

Procarbazine is a methylhydrazine which suppresses mitosis by prolonging interphase and causing a high percentage of chromatid breaks. It is effective in the treatment of Hodgkin's disease.

L-Asparaginase is an enzyme which breaks down the amino acid L-asparagine to aspartic acid and ammonia. It therefore reduces the body pool of asparagine on which some neoplastic cells may be dependent. It is derived from cultures of *Escherichia coli* and of *Erwinia carotovera*, and is particularly effective in inducing remissions in acute lymphatic leukaemia in children, although resistance to it rapidly develops.

Hormones

Prednisolone is effective in many malignant disorders of the reticulo-endothelial system. It suppresses activity of lymphoid tissue and may be associated with an increase in cells of the myeloid and platelet series. In addition, it may reverse the bleeding tendency and inhibit the auto-agglutination which is often found in these disorders.

Oestrogens, androgens and progestogens are used in the treatment of neoplasia in organs which are normally under the influence of the sex hormones, such as the breast, ovary, uterus and prostate.

Thyroid hormone, administered as thyroxine or desiccated thyroid extract, may cause regression of differentiated carcinoma of the thyroid and its metastases.

Radioactive compounds

Radioactive iodine (^{131}I) is concentrated in thyroid tissue and is used for the detection and treatment of inoperable thyroid carcinoma and its metastases. Only about 15 per cent of tumours are sufficiently well differentiated to concentrate the iodine, however, and so its effectiveness is limited to relatively few patients.

Radioactive gold (^{123}Au) is used to inhibit effusions in serous cavities such as the pleura and peritoneum.

Radioactive phosphorous (^{32}P) accumulates in haemopoietic tissue, producing a reduction in red and white cell counts and it has been used, therefore, in the treatment of polycythaemia.

Cytotoxic activity and the cell cycle

There is experimental evidence from the action of cytotoxic drugs on mouse leukaemia that they may be classified according to their predominant effect on the cell cycle. Cells not actively dividing are said to be resting in the Go state. In the actively dividing cell, the mitosis or M phase is followed by the G₁ interphase; then follows the DNA synthetic or S phase; finally the G₂ interphase before the next M phase. In the mouse leukaemia model, high dose mustine acts non-specifically on dividing and resting cells. Methotrexate, cytosine arabinoside and the vinca alkaloids only kill cells in their proliferating phase and then only at certain stages of the cell cycle. Chlorambucil, cyclophosphamide, flurouracil, busulphan, and the antibiotic cytotoxic agents kill only proliferating cells, but throughout their cell cycle. *Cycle specific* drugs are those that can destroy proliferating cells throughout the generation cycle; *phase specific* drugs affect only one or more phases of the cycle. The relevance of this classification to human oncology is not yet established.

19

Antimicrobial drugs

Modern antimicrobial therapy began in 1935 with the publication by Domagk of the results of a successful trial of an azo dye, Prontosil, in the treatment of erysipelas. The development of other related compounds led to the introduction of potent sulphonamides into clinical practice, and a dramatic reduction in the mortality from puerperal fever immediately followed. These compounds must be distinguished from antibiotics which, by definition, are substances produced by micro-organisms antagonistic to the growth of others in high dilution. The first antibiotic to be used in man was penicillin (in 1940), following the work of Chain and Florey on an extract of cultures of a mould, *Penicillium notatum*. Since this time many clinically-useful antibiotics have been isolated from bacteria from the most unlikely of sources, e.g. cephalosporins were first isolated from a mould grown from a sewage outfall in Sardinia.

Mode of action
It is usual to divide antibacterial drugs into those which are bactericidal, i.e. able to kill the bacteria, and those which are bacteriostatic i.e. preventing their growth, but not killing them. Subsequent destruction of bacteria following treatment with a bacteriostatic drug is brought about by natural defence reactions. This division can be important in practice, for antagonism can occur between drugs from one group and those from the other. Some drugs are bacteriostatic in low concentrations and bactericidal at higher concentrations.

Antimicrobials produce their effect by interfering with one or more vital metabolic pathways in the organism.

(a) *Inhibition of folic acid production.* Unlike man, bacteria synthesize their own folic acid, and this substance is essential as a coenzyme for the normal production of nucleotides required for cell division. Sulphonamides have a structural similarity to *p*-aminobenzoic acid, which is a precursor of folic acid. The drug competes with this precursor and is preferentially incorporated into

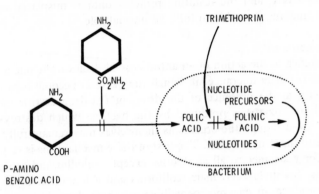

Fig. 20 Sites of action of sulphonamides and trimethoprim.

the folic acid molecule (Fig. 20). The resulting compound is inactive, and bacteria fail to divide.

Trimethoprim, acts at a different point in the folic acid pathway, selectively inhibiting the bacterial enzyme dihydrofolate reductase. Combination of this compound with sulphamethoxazole produces a preparation with potent antibacterial actions (co-trimoxazole).

(b) *Inhibition of cell wall synthesis*. The bacterial cell wall is synthesized from a variety of amino acids, nucleotides and mucopeptides, and a number of points in the complex metabolic pathway can be inhibited by antibiotics. Penicillins act at the final, stage of cross-linking of mucopeptide molecules, and lead to the production of a weak cell wall, resulting in subsequent lysis of the cells (i.e. a bactericidal effect). Other antibiotics, e.g. bacitracin, vancomycin and cycloserine, act at earlier stages of the pathway, and have a different spectrum of activity.

(c) *Inhibition of protein synthesis*. Bacteria, like other cells, manufacture proteins from amino acids in the cytoplasmic ribosomes. Messenger RNA specifies the sequence of amino acids for the protein being produced, and transfer RNA transfers the appropriate amino acids as they are required. Antibiotics can disturb this process in a number of ways. Chloramphenicol inhibits the transfer of the growing peptide chain to the amino acid which has been newly attached to the ribosome. Tetracyclines interfere with the linkage necessary for this transfer. Macrolides and lincomycin disturb the translocation of the messenger RNA which normally brings the next codon opposite the amino acid attachment site. Finally, streptomycin and the other aminoglycosides attach themselves to the ribosome and cause misreading of information supplied by messenger RNA, and the resulting protein contains misplaced amino acids, making it unable to fulfil its normal role.

Drug resistance

Resistance to the action of an antimicrobial drug can be one of two types, (a) drug-tolerance, in which the bacteria become capable of growing in the presence of the drug, or (b) drug-destruction, in which an enzyme is produced by the bacteria which destroys the drug, even though the organisms themselves may remain fully sensitive to the drug's action. The first of these mechanisms is responsible for resistance to all antibiotics except penicillin and cephalosporins. Staphylococci, many coliforms and a few other organisms can produce an enzyme, penicillinase, which degrades penicillin, although newer compounds have been synthesized which are stable to the action of the enzyme. A cephalosporinase can be produced by some bacterial species. There is usually a cross-resistance with chemically related drugs, e.g. when resistance has been acquired to one tetracycline, other members of this group will be ineffective also.

The development of a resistant strain is explained either by the selective growth of a small number of naturally-resistant bacteria or by the occurrence of spontaneous mutation, giving rise to drug-tolerant organisms. The resistant bacteria become dominant as the drug-sensitive ones are destroyed. Other factors may sometimes be involved, such as transmission of the ability to produce penicillinase from one organism to another by a phage, or transference of plasmids (extrachromosomal genetic particles) from one species to another. This latter mechanism is known to account for the frequent possession of drug-resistance by enterobacteria which have never been exposed to the drug. This is often termed 'infectious' resistance.

Principles of treatment

The object of treatment with an antimicrobial drug is to produce at the site of infection a concentration of the drug which is higher than the minimal effective concentration, and which is maintained at the level until the organisms have been eliminated. Failure to meet these requirements encourages the development of resistance. If the drug is being given for a systemic infection it is preferable to give it parenterally if there is any doubt about its absorption (e.g. penicillin).

The frequency of administration is determined by the half-life of the drug in the serum. When renal and hepatic function are normal the standard dose intervals for a particular drug can be adhered to, but sometimes it is necessary to modify them. For example, the liver of the neonate is unable to metabolize many drugs adequately during the first month or so of its life, and this accounts for the 'grey baby' syndrome which developed when premature infants were given prophylactic chloramphenicol. Aminoglycoside antibiotics are almost entirely eliminated in the urine, so that impairment of renal function will cause accumulation of the drug, with subsequent 8th nerve damage, if normal doses are given. In this instance frequent measurement of the serum concentration of the drug by bioassay is essential, especially in the first few days of treatment until a plateau level has been reached. Computer programmes have been written to predict the steady-state level from the kinetics of a single dose, but tables have been published to guide the clinician who lacks this sophisticated help.

The choice of drug for a particular infection is based (a) on the clinical picture (in some infections, e.g. syphilis, the causative organism is invariably sensitive to a particular antibiotic), (b) on the bacteriological diagnosis (which is more often the case, as many infections, e.g. pneumonia, can be caused by one of several organisms), and (c) *in vitro* sensitivity tests. With any one organism there may be a choice of several antimicrobial drugs, and guidance by sensitivity tests can be invaluable in these circumstances. It is usually necessary, however, to start treatment before bacteriological reports are available, and prediction about the type of organism and its sensitivity must be made. Factors such as the cost and potential toxicity of a drug must be taken into account when deciding between several different treatments to which the organisms are equally sensitive. A number of deaths are caused each year by sensitivity to antibiotic drugs, especially penicillins. In addition, there is a considerable morbidity, which is less easy to assess, produced by their toxic actions. It is indefensible when these reactions occur in a patient treated with a powerful drug for a trivial infection, or when the infection (e.g. a common cold) did not justify antibiotic treatment in the first place. Greater discrimination in the use of these drugs would also delay the acquisition of resistance, a problem which has grown almost as rapidly as the number of available drugs has grown.

In general, narrow-spectrum antibiotics are preferable to broad-spectrum agents which, by suppressing commensal bacteria, may encourage, superinfection with resistant organisms, particularly fungi such as *Candida albicans*.

Most infections are successfully treated with a single drug, but occasionally combined treatment is justified. This has two main purposes, (a) to increase bactericidal potency by a synergic effect, and (b) to prevent the development of bacterial resistance. These principles are exemplified by the management of tuberculosis with combinations of two or even three drugs. It is acceptable to combine a bacteriostatic drug with another bacteriostat, or one bactericidal drug with another, but drugs with a different type of action should not be mixed because antagonism may occur. Bactericidal antibiotics (e.g. penicillin) produce their effect on multiplying bacteria, and the presence of a bacteriostatic drug (e.g. tetracycline) will prevent this action.

The route of administration of an antimicrobial drug depends upon its physicochemical nature and on the site of infection to be treated. Streptomycin, for example, is strongly basic and poorly absorbed, and it must therefore be given by injection for systemic infections. A related drug, neomycin, is frequently given orally, however, for bowel infections. Local infections, e.g. conjunctivitis, can be treated by local administration of drugs, but allergy can result from repeated use, particularly of penicillins. Abscesses, e.g. a tuberculous abscess in the lung or empyema, may be walled-off with fibrous tissue which is poorly penetrated by antibiotics, and may have to be treated surgically or by local injection of the drug.

When antibiotics are given in combination the two drugs should not be mixed in the same syringe unless it is known that they are compatible. Precipitation of one drug by a change in pH is a particular hazard. Similarly, a drug given by intravenous infusion should never be added to blood or amino acid solutions. They should be given separately in dextrose or saline, as the manufacturers recommend.

Synthetic Antimicrobials

Sulphonamides

The development of the sulphonamides has produced, in addition to a large number of antibacterial compounds, several clinically useful antidiabetic drugs and a carbonic anhydrase inhibitor with diuretic and anticonvulsant properties (acetazolamide). Those with antimicrobial actions have a wide spectrum of activity covering both Gram-positive and Gram-negative bacteria, with a few exceptions. Strepococci (except *Strep. faecalis*), pneumococci, gonococci and menigococci are highly sensitive, although resistance was acquired early by some species when sulphonamides were widely used, especially gonococci. Resistant meningococci have only recently been reported. Sulphonamides now have a rather restricted use, but remain valuable drugs in urinary tract infections, meningococcal meningitis and bowel infections. The development of resistance is the result of a mutation which produces a folic acid synthetase less sensitive to the action of the drug.

Since the introduction of these compounds the aims of further development have been to produce more potent antibacterial derivatives, which reached a peak with the synthesis of sulphathiazole and sulphadiazine, and to produce compounds whose pharmacokinetics suited them to specific uses. For example, some drugs are rapidly absorbed and rapidly excreted in the urine, sometimes by tubular secretion, making them suitable for use as urinary antiseptics. Other compounds are more slowly excreted and maintain a therapeutic serum level for much longer after a single dose. This property makes them more suitable for the treatment of systemic infections as the antibacterial effect is more constant despite longer dose intervals. Some drugs are absorbed little, if at all, and are suitable for treating bowel infections. These differences are summarized in Table 17.

Sulphonamides are conjugated in the liver to form acetyl derivates, which are excreted in the urine. They lack antibacterial actions. The proportions of parent compound to acetyl-derivative in the urine varies from one drug to another, and this is important in determining potency in urinary infections. The solubility of drug or metabolite in urine is low with some drugs, especially sulphathiazole, sulphadiazine and sulphamerazine. This can lead to crystal formation in the renal tubules, causing haematuria and blockage of tubules or ureter. This problem is minimized either by giving alkali with the drug, as solubility is increased in an alkaline urine, or by administration of a triple mixture (usually a preparation combining sulphadiazine, sulphathiazole and sulphamerazine).

Acetylation of sulphadimidine, like that of isoniazid, is bimodally distributed, i.e. some subjects are slow acetylators, and others are fast. As there is corresponsence between the rate of acetylation of these two drugs, sulphadimidine has been used to identify slow acetylators before starting isoniazid therapy.

Sulphonamides are bound to plasma proteins to a variable extent, the most highly bound being sulphamethizole and sulphamethoxypyridazine, which are over 90 per cent bound. This explains the occurrence of kernicterus of newborn whose mothers have received sulphonamide drugs shortly before delivery. Displacement of

Table 17

Absorption	Good	Good	Good	Good	v. poor
	Short acting	Medium acting	Long acting	Non-absorbed
Distribution	Wide	Wide	Wide	Wide	
Half-life	<6 hours	Up to 20 hours	Up to 40 hours		
Excretion	Rapid	Moderate	Slow		
Frequency of administration	4–6 hourly	12 hourly	Once daily		
Uses	Systemic infections Urinary infections Eye infections	Systemic infections	Systemic infections	Bowel infections	
Examples	Sulphadimidine Sulphafurazole Sulphathiazole Sulphamethizole Sulphacetamide (eye drops only)	Sulphamethoxazole Sulphadiazine	Sulphamethoxydiazine Sulphamethoxypyridazine Sulphadimethoxine Sulphaphenazole Sulphametopyrazine[a] Sulphadimethoxine[a]	Succinylsulphathiazole Phthalysulphathiazole Sulphasalazine[b]	

[a] A single dose gives a therapeutic serum level for a week.
[b] Compound of sulphapyridine and salicyclic acid, used in ulcerative colitis.

bilirubin from its binding sites leads to excessive transfer across the poorly formed blood-brain barrier, and staining of the basal ganglia (kernicterus) occurs, causing a disturbance of their function.

In addition to the adverse effects already mentioned, sulphonamides can produce hypersensitivity reactions, including skin rashes, polyarteritis and the Stevens-Johnson syndrome. Leukopenia occasionally occurs, and haemolytic anaemia from production of methaemoglobin is seen in patients who have a deficiency of glucose-6-phosphate dehydrogenase in their erythrocytes.

Trimethoprim
Trimethoprim has a strongly synergic effect with sulphonamides (Fig. 15) and a combination of trimethoprim with sulphamethoxazole was first introduced as a broad spectrum antibacterial preparation in 1969. Sulphamethoxazole was chosen for the combination as it has a serum half-life similar to that of trimethoprim. The combination has the official name co-trimoxazole, and contains one part of trimethoprim to five parts of the sulphonamide. This proportion produces serum levels of approximately 1:20 in favour of the sulphonamide, and this ratio is optimum for antibacterial effect against most species.

More recently, a combination of trimethoprim and sulphadiazine has been introduced under the approved name, co-trimazine. The reasoning behind this alternative combination is that a much larger proportion of sulphadiazine is excreted in an unchanged and active form in the urine and co-trimazine therefore has an advantage over co-trimoxazole in urinary tract infections. Furthermore, the half-lifes of sulphadiazine and its metabolite increase in renal failure to a similar extent to that of trimethoprim, whereas the metabolite of sulphamethoxazole accumulates and can cause toxicity.

Whereas trimethoprim and the sulphonamide drug are bacteriostatic when given alone, the combination may be bactericidal. In addition, the spectrum of activity of the combinations is wider than that of the constituent drugs alone, and they can be used in infections where a broad spectrum antibiotic is indicated, e.g. a mixed respiratory infection. Trimethoprim is largely excreted unchanged in the urine, and the combination preparations are therefore very effective in urinary tract infections, particularly when complicated by renal tissue involvement. However in uncomplicated acute urinary tract infection, trimethoprim alone is probably as effective as a combination of trimethoprim and a sulphonamide, and is less likely to provoke unwanted effects. Whether a large increase in resistance to trimethoprim will occur if it is used extensively alone is uncertain.

Co-trimoxazole has been successfully used also for treating gonorrhoea, the causative organism of which has become sensitive to sulphonamides again since these compounds have fallen from favour. Typhoid fever has been successfully treated with the combination.

Adverse effects have been comparatively few, although nausea was common when higher doses were being used in early trials. Although mammalian dihydrofolate reductase is 50 000 times less sensitive to trimethoprim than is its bacterial counterpart, long-term co-trimoxazole therapy can produce neutropenia, thrombocytopenia and even aplastic anaemia. Folate-deficient patients with megaloblastic changes are particularly sensitive. Large doses have caused teratogenic effects in rats, and therefore its use cannot be commended during pregnancy.

Urinary antiseptics

A number of compounds are active against the common urinary pathogens, are excreted in high concentration in the urine, and because of their rapid excretion have little systemic antibacterial effect. These drugs are labelled 'urinary antiseptics'.

Hexamine mandelate. This is a compound of hexamine and mandelic acid. The former liberates formaldehyde in an acid medium, and this substance is inhibitory to all species of bacterium. To be effective the pH of the urine should be kept below 5·5, which is not easy to do in practice. Mandelic acid is combined with hexamine with this aim in mind, for it is excreted unchanged and is itself inhibitory to bacteria. However, it is seldom adequate to maintain urinary acidity without the addition of other acidifying agents such as ammonium chloride, ascorbic acid or methionine. The latter agent increases the output of urinary sulphates, but by its effect on trans-sulphuration reactions it can cause vitamin B_6 deficiency. Hexamine will release formaldehyde in the stomach and therefore has to be enteric-coated.

Urine infected with urea-splitting organisms, e.g. *Proteus*, cannot effectively be acidified, and it may be necessary to use a drug which is active in an alkaline urine, such as an aminoglycoside antibiotic.

Nitrofurantoin. This drug is particularly effective in *Esch. coli* infections, but is not active against *Pseudomonas* or some *Proteus* strains. It is most effective in an acid urine, into which it is rapidly excreted and to which it imparts a fluorescent yellow colour. Only about one third of the oral dose can be recovered from the urine, the remainder being broken down in the tissues. Adequate antibacterial levels are reached in the kidney interstitium and the drug can be used for treating acute pyelonephritis.

Adverse effects include gastrointestinal upsets, allergic reactions and peripheral eosinophilia. Peripheral neuropathy, not responsive to vitamin B therapy, occurs with prolonged or excessive therapy, particularly in the presence of impaired renal function, but is usually reversible. Renal function should be investigated before prescribing a prolonged course. Haemolytic anaemia has been reported in patients with glucose-6-phosphate dehydrogenase deficiency.

Nalidixic acid. The spectrum of activity of this compound is similar to that of nitrofurantoin. It is rapidly excreted in the urine mainly as metabolites, some of which are inactive. Resistance readily occurs, lessening its usefulness for treating chronic infections or for long-term suppressive therapy. Raised intracranial pressure has accompanied its use in children.

Cinoxacin is chemically related to nalidixic acid and has the advantage that it needs to be given only twice daily rather than four times daily.

Antitrichomonal drugs

Metronidazole is the only commonly used trichomonacide and has been successfully used in treating giardiasis and amoebiasis. It is also active against *Bacteriodes* species and is used in the treatment of infections of the alimentary tract (including the mouth, where Vincent's infection is one of them), and also for systemic *Bacteriodes* infections. It is well absorbed orally and rectally, and is excreted largely unchanged in the urine. Adverse effects include nausea, a metallic taste in the mouth, furry tongue, rashes and a disulfiram-like flushing and hypotension. (Disulfiram is a drug which blocks alcohol metabolism at the stage of acetaldehyde formation, and is used in treating alcoholism.)

Synthetic drugs for tuberculosis

Prolonged treatment with antimicrobial drugs is necessary to establish a cure in tuberculosis. Because the organisms readily acquire resistance to a single agent, combinations of drugs are used. The traditional combination has been streptomycin, p-aminosalicylic acid and isoniazid, but the former two compounds are now normally replaced by rifampicin, ethambutol or thioacetazone. In 1976, the British Thoracic Association recommended nine months chemotherapy with rifampicin plus isoniazid, with ethambutol added for the first two months, as the preferred treatment of pulmonary tuberculosis in Britain. Only the synthetic drugs are considered here. Alternative antibiotics to streptomycin are considered on page 246.

Isoniazid. Isonicotinic acid hydrazide (INAH) has been successfully used in treating tuberculosis since 1952. It combines high potency, cheapness (an important factor in developing countries) and low toxicity. Taken orally it is well absorbed and penetrates effectively into tissues and the cerebrospinal fluid. About 60 per cent of Caucasians are slow inactivators (by hepatic acetylation), and this trait is genetically determined, probably by a recessive gene. Adverse effects are confined mainly to this group, but high dosage over a prolonged period is necessary to produce these effects. Peripheral neuropathy, responding to pyridoxine treatment, is the most serious. Pyridoxine should be given prophylactically when high doses are administered. Other adverse effects, such as restlessness, insomnia, muscle twitching and difficulty in starting micturition also occur.

Ethambutol. This is a powerful drug without cross-resistance. It is well absorbed orally and about half the dose is excreted unchanged in the urine. In renal insufficiency a reduction in dose is necessary. In general it is well tolerated but it is toxic to the optic nerve, producing either central or periaxial retrobulbar neuritis. Evidence of decreased visual acuity or red-green colour discrimination should be sought at regular ophthalmological assessment. Peripheral neuritis may also occur.

Para-aminosalicylic acid (PAS). This drug, usually given as the sodium salt, is well absorbed, widely distributed and rapidly excreted. Up to 15 g daily are required and this may produce a sodium overload in patients with incipient heart failure. In these patients the calcium or potassium salt should be substituted. Gastrointestinal upsets and allergic reactions are common, usually beginning a few weeks after starting treatment. The latter usually present as fever and skin rashes, but lymphadenopathy, hepatosplenomegaly, transient lung shadows and eosinophilia also occur. Sodium PAS is usually given in cachets combined with isoniazid.

Thioacetazone. As a cheap alternative to PAS, this drug has become popular in developing countries. It is as effective as PAS, and can be given with isoniazid as a single daily dose. It produces adverse-effects more frequently, particularly in doses of about 150 mg/day.

Ethionamide. Like isoniazid, this compound is a derivative of nicotinic acid, although cross-resistance with isoniazid is not shown. It is a potent bactericide, but has a high incidence of adverse effects, particularly on the gastrointestinal tract. Prothionamide is similar, although less toxic. These drugs are useful when resistance has been acquired by the organisms to the standard drugs.

Pyrazinamide. This is another nicotinic acid derivative of moderate potency. Hepatotoxicity is the chief risk, and serum transaminase enzymes should be estimated frequently during its administration.

Antibiotics

Penicillins

No satisfactory method has been developed of synthesizing the penicillin nucleus (6-aminopenicillanic acid) for commercial production. It is obtained by large-scale culture of a high yielding strain of *Penicillium*. Phenylacetic acid is added to the medium in order to encourage the production of benzyl side chains, giving benzyl penicillin (penicillin G). This side chain can be removed enzymatically for the manufacture of newer semi-synthetic penicillins with alternative side chains.

Benzyl penicillin. As the pottassium salt this is known as 'soluable' or 'crystalline' penicillin. It is highly soluble but is unstable at acid pH, and for this reason is poorly active by mouth. After intramuscular injection it is rapidly absorbed. It diffuses well into the tissues but is not found in very high concentration in the CSF. In meningitis the concentration rises higher, owing to fluid exudation, but intrathecal injection is often used to supplement the levels, even though distribution throughout the CSF is incomplete.

Urinary excretion of benzyl penicillin is extremely rapid, being largely by tubular secretion. In order to maintain an effective serum level large doses have to be given at frequent intervals. In early clinical trials this severely hampered treatment as only small amounts of penicillin were available, and the drug had to be re-extracted from the patient's urine. Tubular secretion can be inhibited by concurrent administration of probenecid, and this will produce higher serum levels for the same dose. In practice this is seldom necessary except in some cases of streptococcal endocarditis.

An alternative method of prolonging the duration of action has been employed in preparations whose absorption from the site of injection is delayed. Procaine penicillin, an equimolar compound of penicillin and procaine, is administered as a suspension of crystals which have low solubility. Effective levels can be maintained by a single daily injection. Benethamine penicillin and benzathine penicillin are even less soluble and produce a low concentration in the serum for 4–5 days and several weeks respectively. It is important to bear in mind, however, that the serum level achieved is determined by a dynamic equilibrium between rate of absorption and rate of excretion, and as the latter is unchanged the levels are inevitably considerably lower with long-acting preparations. This makes them unsuitable for acute infections.

Benzyl penicillin is active against most Gram-positive and some Gram-negative organisms, but the latter tend to be less sensitive. Haemolytic streptococci and pneumococci are always highly sensitive and because it has a powerfully bactericidal action, benzyl penicillin remains the drug of choice in these infections. Staphylococci and gonococci are also highly sensitive but resistant strains have become so widespread that alternative drugs are usually preferable unless the results of *in vitro* sensitivity tests are to hand. Resistance is usually the result of penicillinase production by the bacteria, and this may interfere also with the effect of the drug on other organisms present at the site of the infection which are intrinsically sensitive to the drug. Benzyl penicillin is to be preferred for treating meningococcal infections, for the organism is now often resistant to sulphonamides. Benzyl penicillin or a longer-acting preparation are still the treatment of choice for syphilis.

Benzyl penicillin has three main disadvantages, (a) it is destroyed by gastric acid, (b) it is inactivated by penicillinase and (c) its spectrum of activity is too restricted. Efforts to overcome these defects have been successful.

Acid-resistant penicillins. There are four acid-resistant penicillins in common use for oral administration: (a) phenoxymethyl penicillin (penicillin V); (b) phenoxyethyl penicillin (phenethicillin); (c) phenoxypropyl penicillin (propicillin); and (d) phenoxybenzyl penicillin (phenbenicillin).

The first of these is produced by the addition of phenoxyacetic acid to the culture medium, whereas the remaining three are semisynthetic. Although the semisynthetic drugs are better absorbed they are also more highly protein bound, and the serum level of free drug differs little between these preparations. They are excreted rapidly and should therefore be given 4–6 hourly. Gram-negative organisms are less sensitive to these penicillins than to benzyl penicillin.

Penicillinase-resistant penicillins. These penicillins are semisynthetic, and have side chains which protect the β-lactam ring of the penicillin nucleus from the actions of penicillinase (β-lactamase). However, they are much less active than benzyl penicillin against bacterial species which do not produce penicillinase.

Flucloxacillin is the most satisfactory of these for it is acid-resistant and is therefore active orally. Its absorption is better than that of cloxacillin, which must be given by intramuscular injection in the initial treatment of an acute infection. Both drugs are extensively protein-bound in the serum, which reduces their effectiveness.

Methicillin, the first penicillinase-resistant drug to be discovered, is less satisfactory. It must be injected as it is not acid-resistant, and it is much less active than cloxacillin against *Staph aureus* and group A haemolytic streptococci. It is rapidly excreted in the urine and injections must be given every 4–6 hours. It is less protein-bound than cloxacillin.

Broad-spectrum penicillins. Ampicillin, a semisynthetic drug with an α-aminobenzyl side chain, has almost as much activity against Gram-positive organisms as benzyl penicillin, but much greater activity against Gram-negative, particularly *H.influenzae, Proteus mirabilis, Esch. coli* and pathogenic enterobacteria. It is not penicillinase-resistant, but it is acid-resistant and gives good blood levels when administered orally. It is of particular use in urinary infections and mixed respiratory infections but it should not be used in streptococcal pharyngitis in which simple penicillins are as effective, less expensive and less likely to produce a skin rash. As it is active against meningococci, pneumococci and *H.influenzae* it is valuable in meningitis, particularly when the organism cannot be isolated. However, resistance to the latter organism has been reported, and therefore chloramphenicol might be a better choice in life-threatening *Haemophilus* infections. Although excreted largely in the urine, its concentration in bile is high and this makes it suitable for treating typhoid carrier state. Amoxicillin is similar to ampicillin, but is better absorbed. and is therefore given in lower dosage. Pivampicillin and talampicillin are esters of ampicillin which are hydrolysed in the intestinal mucosa and portal system to the parent compound. They are also better absorbed. They cannot, however, be given parenterally as the unhydrolysed compound may be toxic.

Carbenicillin differs from ampicillin in being much more active against strains of Gram-negative bacteria, particularly *Ps. aeruginosa* and *Proteus*. High serum levels must be maintained, however, to eradicate these infections, and as the drug is rapidly excreted in the urine large frequent parenteral doses are required. Combination with gentamicin for severe Gram-negative infections has been recommended. Ticarcillin is a newer alternative without obvious advantages. Carfecillin is an ester of carbenicillin which can be given orally for treating urinary infections. Its concentration in serum is too low for it to be effective in systemic infections.

Mecillinam. This is an amidino-penicillin, having the side chain joined to the β-lactam ring by a β-amidino group. It acts only on one enzyme of the bacterial cell wall. It has a novel spectrum of activity in being particularly effective against Gram negative rods, e.g. *E.coli*, *Klebsiella* species, *Enterobacter* species, *Salmonellae* and some *Proteus* species. However, *Pseudomonas aeruginosa* and *Haemophilus influenzae* are resistant. It is inactive against Gram positive organisms. It should be reserved for treatment of resistant Gram negative urinary tract infections. Pivmecillinam is an ester of mecillinam which is hydrolysed on absorption to release mecillinam.

Adverse effects from penicillins. Benzyl penicillin is remarkably non-toxic. The only dose-related adverse effects to be reported on systemic administration are convulsions, nephritis and haemolytic anaemia, but they have only occurred with huge doses given for a long time, or in the presence of renal disease. In contrast, intrathecal administration of doses greater than 20 000 units readily produces convulsions.

Allergic reactions to all penicillins are common, particularly skin rashes. Essentially they can be divided into two types, (a) immediate anaphylactic reactions, probably produced mainly by penicillin breakdown products in the preparation, and (b) delayed serum sickness type of responses, probably caused by hapten formation by the penicilloyl derivative of penicillanic acid. Immediate anaphylactic reactions occur in one in 10 000 to one in 100 000 patients. Although this is rare, it cannot be ignored for penicillins are widely administered, often unnecessarily, and it is a disaster when a fatal reaction occurs in a young person. It is important to inquire routinely about any previous adverse effects to penicillin before administering it to a patient.

Ampicillin rashes occur very frequently, usually appearing several days after starting treatment, or even after stopping it, and have a characteristic erythematous or maculopapular appearance. They occur in almost every patient who has infectious mononucleosis and who receives ampicillin for the accompanying sore throat. Ampicillin rashes do not necessarily indicate allergy to penicillins in general.

Local application of penicillins, e.g. eye drops, readily produces sensitization. This probably does not apply to penicillin chewing-gum, which has been popular for treating sore throats. Contact dermatitis in nurses who handle penicillins can be a problem.

Broad-spectrum penicillins taken orally frequently produce diarrhoea by altering the bowel flora.

Cephalosporins

The nucleus of the cephalosporin molecule, 7-aminocephalosporanic acid, has a similar structure to the nucleus of the penicillins, but it differs particularly in having a high degree of resistance to staphylococcal penicillinase. The original substance, cephalosporin C, had only moderate antibacterial activity, but side chain substitution has improved this. The newer preparations described below have a wide spectrum of activity against Gram negative bacteria, including the common pathogens such as *E. coli*, *Klebsiella* species and *Proteus* species. They are not active against *Pseudomonas aeruginosa* or faecal streptococci. Cephalosporins are invaluable in the treatment of severe undiagnosed sepsis and resistant gonorrhoea, urinary tract and chest infections. In the penicillin-allergic patient there is some degree of cross allergenicity and a cephalosporin should therefore be avoided if possible.

Cephalothin was the first to be used clinically, and is highly resistant to penicillinase. However, some Gram-negative bacteria can produce a cephalosporinase (a β-lactamase specific for the cephalosporin molecule rather than the penicillin one). Its spectrum of activity is similar to ampicillin, but staphylococci are invariably sensitive to it no matter how much penicillinase they produce. It must be given by injection.

Cephaloridine has been more widely used than cephalothin in Britain. It differs in having greater antibacterial activity than cephalothin, particularly for streptococci and pneumococci, and in being more stable. It is less resistant, however, to penicillinase, and some strains of straphylococcus which produce large amounts of penicillinase can grow in its presence. Like cephalothin, it is poorly absorbed and has to be given by 6-hourly injection. It is nephrotoxic particularly in patients receiving frusemide. Cephaloridine is nephrotoxic and should be avoided in renal failure. Cephazolin is similar in spectrum to cephaloridine.

Three new injectable cephalosporins, cefuroxime, cefoxitin and cephamandole, have essentially the same spectrum of activity as the older cephalosporins, but the first two are particularly stable to β-lactamase.

Cephalexin is also similar to cephaloridine but its activity is lower. It has the advantage of being well absorbed orally although it is less effective than parenterally-administered cephaloridine in more serious urinary tract and respiratory infections. Cephradine and cefaclor are also available for oral use. The latter is particularly active against *H.influenzae*.

Aminoglycosides

A number of antibiotics have been isolated from various strains of *Streptomyces* which are found in soil. Only a few of these are clinically useful, and their value is limited by toxic effects on the eighth cranial nerve.

Streptomycin was discovered shortly after penicillin was introduced into clinical medicine, and immediately became an important drug because of its activity against the tubercle bacillus, for which it is still the mainstay of treatment. It is bactericidal against many Gram-negative organisms but is less active against Gram-positive.

It is a strong base and remains highly ionized in the gut, and is therefore poorly absorbed. It is normally given intramuscularly as the sulphate. It is eliminated almost entirely by urinary excretion and will accumulate if renal function is impaired. This is of vital importance in elderly patients, in whom ototoxic effects are much more common unless allowance is made for reduced glomerular filtration. The urine concentration of the drug is high and it has a powerful bactericidal effect in Gram-negative urinary infections, especially when the urine is made alkaline. When renal function is normal an effective serum concentration is maintained for 8 hours, and therefore the drug should be given at 8 hourly intervals for acute infections. It is usual to give a single daily dose for tuberculosis.

Bacteria can rapidly acquire resistance to streptomycin, but this can be prevented by combining it with other antibacterial drugs, such as ethambutol and INAH in tuberculosis (p. 234). It is sometimes combined with penicillin for treatment of enterococcal endocarditis. It is effective in plague, tularaemia and brucellosis.

The ototoxicity of the drug is directed mainly towards the vestibular branch of the eighth nerve, whereas dihydrostreptomycin affects the auditory branch. The latter drug is not longer used. When streptomycin has to be given to patients with impaired renal function, therapy should be controlled by microbiological assays of the serum concentration. Streptomycin should not be prescribed without strong bacteriological indications for its use.

Neomycin has a spectrum similar to that of streptomycin, but is more active against staphylococci and *Proteus*. It is not used systemically because it is highly toxic to the auditory branch of the eighth nerve, as well as being nephrotoxic. Resistance is acquired less readily to neomycin than to streptomycin. It has been used for the local treatment of infections, and is a constituent of many skin ointments, nasal sprays, and eye ointments but its value following topical application is doubtful. Like streptomycin, it is little absorbed when given orally and is widely used for suppression of bowel flora pre-operatively and in the prevention of hepatic coma. It should be used in enteritis only if bacteriologically indicated. Its indiscriminate use leads to bacterial resistance and a prolongation of the carrier state. Although it is poorly absorbed, ototoxicity has been reported in patients with poor renal function who have received drugs orally or topically (e.g. following extensive burns).

Kanamycin has a spectrum of activity similar to that of neomycin, but is less ototoxic. It is used for treating tuberculosis in which the bacilli are resistant to standard drugs. It is also used in Gram-negative septicaemia. Deafness can follow its use, and it should be used more circumspectly than streptomycin.

Gentamicin is especially active against *Ps. aeruginosa* and is used in urinary tract infections and septicaemia caused by this organism. In the presence of renal disease, monitoring serum levels is mandatory if vestibular nerve damage is to be avoided. Trough levels should fall below 9 μmol/l (4 μg/ml) but peak levels should exceed 18 μmol/l (8 μg/ml). Staphylococci resistant to streptomycin and neomycin are often sensitive to it. It has been used for local application and for suppression of bowel flora.

Tobramycin is similar to gentamicin. Amikacin is a semisynthetic derivative of kanamycin, and has an advantage over gentamicin and tobramycin in that it is active against many organisms that are resistant to the latter drugs. It should be used only in the treatment of serious gentamicin–resistant Gram negative infections.

Framycetin and paromomycin are alternatives for local application, being too toxic for systemic use.

The ototoxicity of aminoglycosides is potentiated by frusemide and ethacrynic acid.

Chloramphenicol

This compound was originally isolated from a strain of *Streptomyces*, but is now produced synthetically. Its introduction provided one of the first broad spectrum antibiotics which could be administered orally. Its effects are bacteriostatic rather than bactericidal, even in high concentrations. Although it has a wide spectrum of activity it is less effective against Gram-positive organisms than many other antibiotics. Its activity against Gram-negative species, however, makes it a drug of choice in certain situations, but the risk of aplastic anaemia, admittedly small, must be weighed against its potential advantages. The Committee on Safety of Medicines has recommended that it should be used only for treating typhoid fever, *H. influenzae* meningitis, and other infections where no other antibiotic will suffice. Its pre-eminence in typhoid fever has been undoubted, although it now has a challenger in the form of co-trimoxazole, which may prove to be as effective and certainly less toxic. For *H. influenzae* meningitis also, ampicillin has been shown to be equally effective, and this drug may be preferable. In the opinion of many clinicians chloramphenicol still has an important place in treating severe exacerbations of chronic bronchitis or severe pertussis, but its use can seldom be justified in other situations.

Bacterial resistance to chloramphenicol occurs slowly, but is seldom troublesome in countries where it is not widely used. Resistance can be of 'infectious' type among enterobacteria.

Chloramphenicol is well absorbed orally, is largely conjugated in the liver and is excreted mainly as inactive glucuronides in the urine. It diffuses particularly well into the CSF. The capacity to conjugate the drug is inadequate in the first month of life and the accumulation of the parent compound causes the 'grey-baby syndrome' in neonates and premature babies, which is characterized by vasomotor collapse.

Chloramphenicol is toxic to the bone marrow in two ways. First, it causes a dose-related depression that depends upon the inhibition of mitochondrial protein synthesis and which is entirely reversible on withdrawal. The red cell series is primarily involved. This type of toxicity occurs commonly when the dose exceeds 2 g daily for more than 10 days, but it can be predicted by regular blood counts. The second type of toxic effect is a more serious aplasia which is frequently irreversible and ultimately fatal. It is not dose related and probably results from depression of DNA synthesis is stem cells. Although rare (one in 20 000 administrations) it cannot be predicted by regular blood counts.

Tetracyclines

The first of these compounds, chlortetracycline, was introduced in 1948, at the same time as chloramphenicol. It is obtained from a species of *Steptomyces*, and minor changes in its molecule produces two other widely used compounds, tetracycline and oxytet-racycline. The spectrum of activity is similar for each of these compounds and there are only minor differences in their pharmacokinetics.

Like chloramphenicol they are active against a wide variety of organisms, including some viruses and chlamydia. They are bacteriostatic rather than bactericidal, and should not be combined with bactericidal antibiotics such as penicillin. They differ in having useful activity in a number of less common infections, such as brucellosis, tularaemia, leptospirosis, cholera, anthrax, gas gangrene, typhus, Q fever, trachoma, psittacosis, lymphogranuloma venereum and actinomycosis.

They are most commonly prescribed for chronic bronchitis. Acute upper respiratory tract infections and pneumonias should not be treated with tetracycline because many Gram-positive organisms have developed resistance. This is true also of many enterobacteria, in which resistance of the 'infectious' type may occur. Although the use of a broad-spectrum drug in mixed infections seems attractive, the widespread prescription of them for any bacteriologically-undiagnosed infection is causing an increasing problem of resistance, which may eventually severely limit their usefulness.

Tetracylines are slowly and incompletely absorbed, particularly when calcium- or iron-containing preparations are given concurrently, when chelation occurs in the bowel. They are excreted mainly into the urine, but the concentration in bile is moderately high and this prolongs their action by 'enterohepatic' circulation.

Incomplete absorption is responsible for the most troublesome of adverse effects, diarrhoea. This is very common and is probably caused mainly by elimination of normal bowel flora, allowing overgrowth of resistant staphylococci and abnormal enterobacteria. *Candida albicans* can also colonize the bowel, but addition of nystatin to tetracycline preparations does not reduce the incidence of diarrhoea and therefore there is no indication for administering these expensive preparations.

Children under the age of 8 years should, if possible, not be given tetracyclines, for they are deposited in bones and teeth, producing a yellowing of the second dentition. Tetracyclines should also be avoided in pregnancy. Dose-dependent hepatocellular damage can be produced by parenteral administration.

Tetracyclines should not be used in patients known to have renal insufficiency because they accumulate, promote protein breakdown and exacerbate renal failure.

A number of newer tetracyclines have been introduced since the original three were developed, but the advantages they offer are few. Demeclocycline and methacycline have a slightly higher antibacterial activity, are excreted more slowly and therefore can be given 12 hourly rather than 6 hourly. Doxycycline is even more slowly excreted and can be given once daily. Lymecycline, minocycline and clomocycline may be better absorbed, producing less diarrhoea, but this requires confirmation. Pyrrolidinomethyl tetracycline is a highly soluble preparation for parenteral administration.

Macrolides

Erythromycin possesses a spectrum of activity similar to that of penicillin, and has been used chiefly as a substitute for this drug when sensitivity to it occurs. It is bactericidal only in higher concentrations. Bacterial resistance can become a problem, particularly with staphylococci, and addition of a second drug, such as novobiocin, is judicious if this is to be avoided. Combination with penicillin has proved useful for treating *Strep. viridans* endocarditis.

It is moderately well absorbed and can be given as the base, stearate or estolate. The latter is better absorbed and produces higher blood levels than the base, which is not stable to gastric acid. It is excreted in high concentration in the bile and recirculates through the liver. Most of it appears to be broken down in the body, for little can be recovered from the urine.

Diarrhoea is one of the commonest adverse effects, produced by alteration in bowel flora. The estolate can produce dose-independent cholestatic jaundice.

Oleandomycin has a similar spectrum to erythromycin and is less potent. It shares the property of hepatoxicity and appears to have no advantage over erythromycin.

Spiramycin is the least active of these compounds, although this may be compensated by its selective concentration in liver, kidney, spleen and lung.

Peptide antibiotics

These antibiotics are produced primarily by certain strains of bacilli, and comprise a polypeptide chain linked to some other group, e.g. a long chain fatty acid as in the polymyxins.

Bacitracin was first discovered in a culture from an infected wound of a child, Margaret Tracey, after whom the drug was named. It is now rarely used systemically as it is nephrotoxic and other antibiotics are more satisfactory alternatives. It is active mainly on Gram-positive cocci, particularly haemolytic streptococci of group A. It is not absorbed orally and therefore has to be injected for systemic use. It is slowly excreted in the urine, and causes degeneration of the epithelial lining of the convoluted tubules, which can lead to anuria if the drug is continued.

Bacitracin is used mainly for treating infections of the skin, and for this purpose it is often combined with neomycin and polymyxin. It has also been used for preparation of the bowel before surgery.

Polymyxins used in clinical practice are of two types, B and E. The latter was introduced as colistin. Both these compounds are bactericidal primarily against Gram-negative organisms, including many enterobacteria and, most important, *Ps. aeruginosa*. Their main use has been in infections with this latter organism, although this position is now being challenged by newer drugs, particularly gentamicin. They are not absorbed from the gut, and must be given by injection either as the sulphate or sulphomethyl derivatives. The latter are the most popular for they do not cause pain at the site of injection, as do the sulphates, and they produce fewer adverse effects.

Renal tubular damage occurs much less frequently than with bacitracin, and then usually only when there is pre-existing renal damage. Polymyxin E is less nephrotic than B. Numbness and paraesthesiae, particularly of the face, can occur, usually with the sulphates.

As with bacitracin, the polymyxins are used widely for local application to the skin, eyes and ears.

Antibiotics for penicillin-resistant organisms
One of the chief problems which has faced the bacteriologist and clinician ever since the introduction of penicillin is that of resistance, either by production of penicillinase or by mutation yielding a drug-tolerant variant. Staphylococci are notorious in this respect, and many of the antibiotics which have been developed in recent years have been aimed at these organisms. The following drugs are examples of these. They are not used widely, as the newer penicillinase-resistant penicillins and cephalosporins are currently favoured in this situation.

Fusidic acid is unusual in having a steroid structure. It is well absorbed orally as the sodium salt. Natural resistance is rare, but it can develop during treatment. For this reason it is preferable to combine it with penicillin, erythromycin or novobiocin.

Novobiocin was one of the earliest developments against resistant staphylococci and is usually given with erythromycin to delay bacterial resistance, which develops rapidly when it is used alone. It is well absorbed orally, is excreted in high concentration in the bile, and recirculates. Urticarial rashes are particularly common if it is used for more than a week.

Clindamycin, although chemically different from erythromycin, resembles it in its spectrum of activity and shows cross-resistance with it. It is more active and better absorbed than its predecessor, lincomycin. It reaches adequate concentrations in bone and has been used successfully in osteomyelitis. Its major adverse effect is pseudo-membranous colitis and its use should therefore be restricted to staphylococcal bone and joint disease and intra-abdominal sepsis (with an aminoglycoside).

Vancomycin is indicated only in resistant staphylococcal or streptococcal endocarditis and in anti-bacterial associated colitis. It is not absorbed orally and causes tissue necrosis on intramuscular injection, and must therefore be given by intravenous infusion. It is bactericidal, and resistance develops rarely. It can cause deafness if the serum concentration is excessive.

Spectinomycin is reserved for the treatment of penicillin-resistant gonorrhoea.

Antibiotics for resistant tuberculosis
If resistance is developed to the standard drugs used for combined therapy one of the following antibiotics can be of value. Synthetic drugs are discussed on page 234.

Rifampicin is bactericidal and highly active against *Myco. tuberculosis* and staphylococci. It is well absorbed orally and is excreted in the bile. Resistance occurs easily and therefore it should be combined with another drug. It is being used increasingly to replace streptomycin in both initial and maintenance therapy. Rifampicin plus isoniazid plus ethambutol is a satisfactory combination for initial treatment, the latter drug being dropped for maintenance therapy. Rifampicin is expensive and this limits it use in developing countries. Although active against staphylococci, it is reserved for use in tuberculosis. It is a potent liver enzyme inducing agent (p. 23).

Capreomycin is a peptide antibiotic whose main action is against the tubercle bacillus. It is ototoxic and nephrotoxic.

Cycloserine is a broad spectrum antibiotic which is useful in tuberculosis as well as in *Esch. coli* and *Proteus* urinary tract infections. It can produce ataxia, drowsiness and convulsions.

Viomycin resembles streptomycin in its antibacterial activity and toxic effects. The latter, however, are much more frequent, and include giddiness, deafness and renal damage. It must be given by injection.

Antifungal antibiotics

Although some antibacterial antibiotics, e.g. tetracycline, have antifungal activity they are rarely used for this purpose because there are a number of compounds which have specific antifungal activity without much action on bacteria. The three most used antifungal drugs are described below, although a large number of other compounds are available, mainly for local application.

Nystatin, a polyene compound, is now used only for treating local infections caused by *Candida albicans*. Although it acts against other yeast-like fungi it is poorly soluble and not well absorbed from the alimentary tract or from the site of injection. It has been replaced by a much more active polyene compound, amphoterocin B, for systemic infections. Various preparations of nystatin are available for treating infections of the mouth, alimentary tract, vagina and skin.

Amphoterocin B is active against a variety of filamentous and yeast-like fungi. Given intravenously it is effective in the treatment of histoplasmosis, coccidioidomycosis, North American blastomycosis, cryptococcal meningitis and systemic candidiasis. Although highly effective, it is also highly toxic. In therapeutic doses it has nephrotoxic actions, some of which may be permanent, e.g. proliferative changes in the glomeruli. It also causes fever, vomiting anaemic and local thrombophlebitis.

The toxicity of amphoterocin B has lead to a search for alternative compounds which can be used for treating systemic fungal infections. 5-Fluorocytosine is effective in cryptococcal meningitis, but is probably less active than amphoterocin B in systemic candiasis. Clotrimazole is effective in *Candida* infections, particularly when used topically.

Griseofulvin is particularly active against dermatophytes because it is incorporated into the keratin of skin, nails and hair. Treatment may be necessary for up to 2 years in order to completely eliminate nail infections with *Trichophyton*. Its absorption has been improved by decreasing the particle size of oral preparations. Its absorption is impaired by phenobarbitone treatment, and a higher dose should be given to patients receiving long-term barbiturates, e.g. for epilepsy.

Antiviral drugs

The development of clinically-useful antiviral drugs has been slow because of several fundamental problems. Viruses gain entrance to body cells and replicate by distorting normal synthetic processes of the cells. For an agent to suppress viral replication it would first of all have to penetrate into the host cell, and then inhibit the enzymatic processes producing viral nucleic acids and proteins without affecting those of the cell. An even more fundamental difficulty is the fact that the peak rate of growth of the virus is usually over before clinical signs of infection appear, and therefore drug treatment is more suited to prophylaxis than to use in an established infection.

Amantadine blocks the entry of virus particles into cells, but this effect is not powerful. Clinical trials of this compound as a prophylactic drug in influenza have shown variable results, but the duration and severity of the infection seems to be reduced. A more successful application is in the treatment of Parkinsonism (p. 70).

Idoxuridine is a thymidine analogue which inhibits the utilization of thymidine in DNA synthesis. This interferes with the replication of herpes viruses. Continuous topical application of 40 percent idoxuridine in dimethyl-sulphoxide is effective in skin lesions caused by varicella zoster virus. It has been little used systemically because of its likely effects on DNA synthesis in the normal cell, but it appears to have been a life-saving measure when given intravenously to a few patients with herpes simplex encephalitis.

Vidarabine is a purine analogue with activity against herpes viruses; it has a preferential effect on virus as opposed to cellular DNA synthesis. In immunosuppressed patients with shingles it has been shown to reduce pain but its effect is probably small.

Acyclovir is an acyclic nucleoside analogue which is preferentially absorbed by herpes-infected cells where it is phosphorylated by virally specified thymidine kinase into an active substance which inhibits viral DNA polymerase up to thirty times more than cellular DNA polymerase. Theoretically, it should be relatively nontoxic, and given systemically in serious virus infections promising results have been claimed.

Methisazone inhibits pox viruses at a late stage in their maturation. It is of little value in established smallpox but it has been successfully used as a prophylactic agent in smallpox contacts. It appears also to be of value in reducing the severity of vaccinia when it is given on the fourth day after vaccination of patients who are at special risk, e.g. those with eczematous lesions.

Interferons are highly active glycoproteins which are released by cells invaded by virus particles, probably because the virus induces the production of a messenger RNA which acts as a template for interferons. They probably act on cell membrane receptor sites causing intracellular production of proteins which inhibit the translation of viral messenger RNA. Three types of human interferon exist, leucocyte interferon (obtained from buffy-coat lymphocytes which have been exposed to para-influenza virus), fibroblast interferon (derived from fibroblasts induced with synthetic double-stranded RNA) and 'immune' interferon (derived from T lymphocytes exposed to antigens to which they have been sensitised).

Small quantities of interferon have been made available for trial in virus infections. Promising results have been reported in prophylaxis in immunosuppressed patients, in respiratory infections, viral diseases of the eye, herpes zoster and chronic virus infections such as genital warts. Commercial production of larger quantities will allow further evaluation of this potentially valuable therapeutic substance.

20

Anthelmintic drugs

Anthelmintic drugs are an assorted group of compounds which share the property of toxicity to parasitic worms. As helmintic infections are amongst the most common of human diseases, they have wide application. A summary of the drugs available, their mode of action and their applications is given in Table 18.

For the roundworms, *Enterobius vermicularis* and *Ascaris lumbricoides*, and for the hookworm, *Ancylostoma duodenale*, pyrantel pamoate is an effective drug. In *Enterobius vermicularis* infestations, however, mebendazole is equally effective. Both of these drugs have the advantage that single doses are curative. Infestation with the new world hookworm, *Necator americanus*, is best treated with tetrachlorethylene rather than pyrantel pamoate.

Strongyloides stercoralis, which can become disseminated, can be eradicated only with thiabendazole therapy. The nematode, *Trichuris trichuria*, is usually eliminated by mebendazole.

When roundworms invade tissues; e.g. visceral larva migrans caused by the dog roundworm *Toxocara canis*, only non-specific therapy such as systemic anti-inflammatory drugs and corticosteroids can be used. In cutaneous larva migrans caused by dog hookworms, however, thiabendazole may destroy the larvae. Only symptomatic therapy can be offered in *Trichinella spiralis* infestations, which can cause severe multisystem inflammatory disease during the migratory phase.

Filarial infections are difficult to manage; diethylcarbamazine is the best available drug, but release of antigens from dead or dying worms may cause systemic reactions which require corticosteroid therapy.

Tapeworms (*Cestodes*) can generally be eliminated by single dose therapy with niclosamide or multi-dose therapy with paromomycin.

Of the fluke infections, those caused by schistosomes are the most serious. Unfortunately, the antimonial compounds used to eliminate *Schistosoma mansoni* and *S. japonicum* are amongst the more toxic of antihelmintic drugs. Niridazole is a drug of first choice in *S. haematobium* infections.

Drug	Mode of action	Absorption	Excretion	Toxicity	Drug of choice in	Other uses
Pyrantel pamoate	Depolarization of myoneural junction by anticholinesterase effect. Paralysis of worm.	Low	90% faeces 10% urine	Neuromuscular blockade in excess.	*Ascaris* *Enterobius*	Hookworms
Mebendazol	Irreversibly inhibits glucose uptake.	Low	90% faeces 10% urine	None known.	*Trichuris* *Enterobius* *Ascaris*	*Ascaris*
Piperazine	Blocks cholinergic receptors. Paralysis of worm.	High	25% metabolized	No serious toxicity.	*Ascaris*	Hookworms *Enterobius*
Thiabendazole	Unknown. Kills larval and encysted forms.	High	10% faeces 90% urine	Anorexia, nausea, dizziness. Hepatotoxic.	*Strongyloides* Cutaneous larva migrans	
Bephenium hydroxynaphthoate	Unknown.	No	Faeces	Nausea, vomiting, diarrhoea.	*Ancylostoma*	*Necator*
Tetrochlorethylene	Reversibly paralyses worm. Interferes with intracellular digestive processes.	High	Metabolized	Nausea, vomiting. CNS effects.	*Necator*	
Niclosamide	Interferes with respiration and blocks glucose uptake.	No	Faeces	None known.	All tapeworms	
Antimonials (antimony potassium tartrate and stibophen)	Inhibit phosphofructokinase.	Used parenterally	Urine	Vomiting, renal tubular damage, arthralgia, bone marrow depression, bradycardia. Hepatotoxic.	Schistosomes (*S. mansoni*–stibophen; *S. japonicum*–antimony potassium tartrate)	*S. mansoni* *S. japonicum*
Niridazole	Inhibits uptake of exogenous glucose.	Complete	Metabolized	Confusion, convulsions. Flattening of T waves in ECG. Haemolysis in G-6-PD deficient subjects.	*Schistosoma haematobium* *Dracunculus medinensis*	
Diethylcarbamazine	Unknown. Renders microfilariae susceptible to phagocytosis.	High	Urine	Headache, myalgia, athralgia, nausea.	All filariae except *Dracunculus medinensis*	
Paromomycin	Unknown.	Low	Faeces	Diarrhoea.	Tapeworms	
Pyrvinium pamoate	Inhibits oxygen uptake and absorption of exogenous glucose.	No	Faeces	Nausea and vomiting.	*Enterobius*	

21

Treatment of poisoning

Poisoning with drugs may be (a) accidental or (b) deliberate as a suicidal attempt or gesture. When a patient is unconscious or semi-conscious from a drug overdosage, the nature of the drug ingested may not be known, but the patient should be treated according to certain general principles which apply irrespective of the active substance responsible.

1. Maintenance of respiration

Respiratory depression occurs with many centrally acting drugs, particularly the barbiturates and other hypnotics. In addition, there may be airways obstruction due to inhalation of vomitus or excessive mucus production. It is therefore important to ensure a clear airway, if necessary by insertion of a cuffed endotracheal tube or even by tracheostomy. If the patient is cyanosed, or in fact, if there is any suspicion of inadequate ventilation, oxygen should be administered in high concentrations, and intermittent positive pressure ventilation should be considered. If facilities are available the minute volume may be measured with a Wright's spirometer and arterial blood gas analysis may be carried out at regular intervals. There is no place for the use of analeptic drugs in overdosage with centrally acting drugs. They have a narrow therapeutic ratio and readily produce convulsions and cardiac dysrhythmias.

2. Maintenance of cardiovascular function

Depression of the vasomotor and cardiac centres may occur with many drugs. In addition, prolonged vomiting or excessive sweating may cause marked fluid depletion and lead to a state of hypotension and shock. This results in increased sympathetic activity with peripheral vasoconstriction and shunting of blood from skin and splanchnic areas to maintain adequate coronary and cerebral perfusion. Inadequate perfusion of the lungs may lead to metabolic acidosis.

The central venous pressure should be measured and if it is

reduced intravenous fluids should be infused cautiously to increase the circulating volume, venous return and cardiac output. This should be delayed, however, if there is a suggestion of incipient renal failure with acute tubular necrosis (see below) and discontinued if signs of fluid excess appear, for example pulmonary oedema. The use of vasoconstrictor agents such as noradrenaline or metaraminol is controversial. On theoretical grounds it is unlikely to be of value because sympathetic tone is already high in most shocked patients and the administration of α-receptor stimulating drugs may further decrease tissue perfusion in organs such as the gut and kidney. If rehydration fails to raise the blood pressure to acceptable levels intravenous hydrocortisone 100 mg should be given and repeated at regular intervals as necessary. Many psychotropic drugs produce cardiac dysrhythmias and cardiac monitoring should, therefore, be employed where possible during the recovery period in all patients. Antidysrhythmic drugs may, however, potentiate the cardiotoxicity of these compounds.

3. Control of pain
Intense pain may occur with poisoning from ingestion of corrosive substances. It should be treated with potent analgesic drugs such as morphine or heroin, repeated as necessary.

4. Control of convulsions
Convulsions may occur in overdosage with central stimulant drugs and antidepressant compounds and also in phenothiazine and Mandrax poisoning in which the epileptic seizure threshold is reduced. They may be controlled by intravenous injection of diazepam. If severe respiratory depression occurs mechanical ventilation should be used.

5. Reduction of absorption
When it is known that the drug concerned has been ingested within four hours of admission to hospital it may be considered reasonable to attempt to prevent further absorption by emptying the patient's stomach or administering activated charcoal which is said to adsorb drugs on to its surface. If the patient is conscious it may be possible to induce emesis by pharyngeal stimulation. The alternative for the unconscious or semiconscious patient is gastric lavage, but this is a potentially dangerous procedure and must be avoided if there is any suspicion that the patient may have taken corrosives or petroleum substances, and in patients known to have upper alimentary disease. After gastric lavage has been carried out purgation may be

induced by means of 50–100 ml of 70 per cent sorbitol solution given via the gastric tube, so emptying the small bowel of its contents of drug and preventing further absorption. If the patient is unconscious and the protective pharyngeal reflexes are depressed, a cuffed endotracheal tube should be inserted before lavage is attempted.

6. Increase rate of drug elimination

(a) *Diuresis.* In the absence of renal impairment, the patient's kidneys provide a better dialysing membrane than any artificial kidney for the elimination of a drug. However, because renal impairment may have been present before the drug ingestion, or if a state of profound hypotension might have induced acute tubular necrosis, the ability of the kidneys to excrete a fluid load should be assessed before attempting to force a diuresis. This may be done by administering intravenously a small volume of 10 or 20 per cent mannitol and observing the urinary output during the next few minutes. If there is a significant increase in urine output, it is reasonable to proceed to force a diuresis. If not, then intravenous infusion of fluids may precipitate left ventricular failure and pulmonary oedema, and other methods of drug elimination must be considered.

When a diuresis is to be produced two factors must be considered, namely its volume and the urinary pH. The relative importance of these factors differs according to the drug under consideration. When the reabsorption of the drug across the renal tubular membrane from the lumen of the tubule into the blood stream is not markedly pH dependent then the only way to modify the rate of excretion is to increase the volume of urine and hence the rate at which it passes through the tubule. This minimizes the time during which reabsorption of the drug may occur.

In the case of weak acids such as salicylic acid, aspirin and phenobarbitone, and weak bases such as amphetamine and ephedrine, which are excreted to a significant extent in the urine, altering the urinary pH may markedly influence the rate of excretion. The excretion of weakly acidic drugs is increased if the urine is made alkaline, usually by intravenous administration of 1/6 molar lactate solution. Conversely that of weakly basic drugs is increased if the urine is made more acid by oral or intravenous administration of ammonium chloride.

The intravenous administration of sufficient volumes of fluid, either dextrose or saline, may be sufficient to provoke and maintain an adequate diuresis, but it is common practice to use a diuretic as well, either an osmotic drug such as mannitol intravenously (for example 100 ml of 10 per cent mannitol diluted in 500 ml normal saline in one hour) or intravenous frusemide 10–20 mg.

(b) *Dialysis.* Peritoneal or haemodialysis may be considered to increase the rate of elimination of a drug when its blood levels are very high and the clinical condition is poor, or where renal insufficiency precludes the use of forced diuresis.

7. Care of the unconscious patient
Routine care of the unconscious patient should be carefully observed, with particular reference to (a) the skin with frequent regular turning and use of a ripple bed, (b) the bladder with catheterization under strict aseptic conditions, (c) the bowels, and (d) toilet to the mouth, nose and eyes. The nutritional state must also be observed, with institution of parenteral feeding if necessary.

8. Psychiatric treatment and assessment
During the recovery phase, the patient may become agitated, distressed or even violent, and may require sedation with intramuscular chlorpromazine. If the poisoning is considered to have been a suicidal attempt or gesture a full psychiatric assessment should be carried out and appropriate treatment instituted.

SPECIFIC MEASURES

In relatively few cases of poisoning specific measures may be indicated *in addition* to the general measures of treatment already discussed.

Narcotics. Narcotic antagonists (p. 118) may be used in patients poisoned with morphine, heroin, pethidine or other narcotics, in order to reduce respiratory depression, naloxone being the drug of choice. Naloxone is also effective in pentazocine overdosage. However, an acute abstinence syndrome may be precipitated if physical dependence has already developed on the narcotic drug.

Monoamine oxidase inhibitors. Overdosage of monoamine oxidase inhibitors may be associated with hyperpyrexia and excitement for which chlorpromazine is the treatment of choice. If marked hypertension is present this should be treated with an α-adrenergic receptor blocking drug such as phentolamine or thymoxamine.

Cyanide. The inhalation of hydrogen cyanide usually causes death within a few minutes, while with oral ingestion of cyanide salts death may be delayed by as much as an hour. There are two treatment regimens: (a) Amyl nitrite should be administered by inhalation every minute while a sodium nitrite solution is prepared. This is then given intravenously followed by sodium thiosulphate. The purpose of the nitrite is to convert haemoglobin to methaemoglobin which competes with cytochrome oxidase for cyanide. The thiosulphate aids detoxication of cyanide to thiocyanate. (b) Intravenous cobalt edetate followed by a strong dextrose solution.

Corrosive mineral acids. These cause corrosion of mucous membranes of the mouth, throat, oesophagus and stomach, with intense pain and circulatory collapse. Glottal oedema may lead to asphyxia. Gastric lavage and emetics must be avoided, but neutralizing and diluting agents such as milk of magnesia or aluminium hydroxide should be given together with large amounts of water. Demulcents such as olive oil, milk, egg whites or melted butter should also be given.

Disinfectants and antiseptics. These substances usually contain cresol or phenol which, like the corrosive acids, produce widespread ulceration of the upper alimentary tract with shock and circulatory collapse. Gastric lavage is dangerous from risk of perforation. Milk and water should be given in large quantities, and the addition of castor oil may minimize absorption.

Carbon monoxide. The patient should be moved from the atmosphere of carbon monoxide immediately, and pure oxygen administered by the best method available. A whole blood transfusion may be useful if given at an early stage of treatment.

Heavy metals. After oral ingestion of large amounts of metallic salts, for example copper or iron, gastric lavage should be carried out with milk followed by administration of demulcents such as egg whites. Chelating agents should then be used, for example BAL (dimercaprol) or penicillamine (p. 202) for copper poisoning, and desferrioxamine or calcium disodium edetate for iron poisoning.

Paracetamol. Overdosage with paracetamol can produce hepatic necrosis which should be treated as in other patients with this condition. If less than ten hours have elapsed since ingestion, oral methionine should be given. Plasma levels should be measured, and if the concentration is above a line drawn between 1300 μmol/l (200 μg/ml) at 4 hours and 460 μmol/l (70 μg/ml) at 10 hours after ingestion then further oral methionine or intravenous cysteamine or N-acetylcysteine are given. These measures appear to be ineffective after 10 hours following ingestion. It appears that paracetamol hepatotoxicity is due to formation of a toxic alkylating intermediate metabolite which, following therapeutic doses of paracetamol, is normally inactivated by conjugation with hepatic glutathione. In overdosage, however, the glutathione stores are depleted and the excess metabolite binds covalently to macromolecules in the hepatocyte wall to cause necrosis. Methionine, cysteamine and N-acetylcysteine probably exert their protective action by donating sulphydril groups to which the toxic metabolite binds in preference to the hepatocyte macromolecules.

Paraquat a weedkiller which after oral ingestion is particularly toxic to the lungs and for which there is no known antidote, binds strongly to Fuller's earth and bentonite. One of these absorbent substances should therefore be administered as soon as possible after paraquat ingestion.

Subject index

Compound index

CHURCHILL LIVINGSTONE MEDICAL TEXTS

Epidemiology in Medical Practice
Second edition
D.J.P. Barker and G. Rose

Pain: Its Nature, Analysis and Treatment
Michael R. Bond

Essentials of Dermatology
J.L. Burton

Essential Ophthalmology
H. Chawla

Notes on Psychiatry
Fifth edition
I.M. Ingram, G.C. Timbury and R.M. Mowbray

Elements of Medical Genetics
Fifth edition
Alan E.H. Emery

Physiology: A Clinical Approach
Third edition
G.R. Kelman

Tumours: Basic Principles and Clinical Aspects
Christopher Louis

Nutrition and its Disorders
Third edition
Donald S. McLaren

The Essentials of Neuroanatomy
Third edition
G.A.G. Mitchell and D. Mayor

Clinical Bacteriology
P.W. Ross

Sexually Transmitted Diseases
Third edition
C.B.S. Schofield

Notes on Medical Bacteriology
J.D. Sleigh and Morag C. Timbury

An Introduction to General Pathology
Second edition
W.G. Spector

Child Psychiatry for Students
Second edition
Frederick H. Stone and Cyrille Koupernik

Introduction to Clinical Endocrinology
Second edition
John A. Thomson

Notes on Medical Virology
Sixth edition
Morag C. Timbury

Immunology: An Outline for Students of Medicine and Biology
Fourth edition
D.M. Weir

Clinical Thinking and Practice: Diagnosis and Decision in Patient Care
H.J. Wright and D.B. MacAdam

LIVINGSTONE MEDICAL TEXTS

Geriatric Medicine for Students
J.C. Brocklehurst and T. Hanley

An Introduction to Clinical Rheumatology
William Carson Dick

A Concise Textbook of Gastroenterology
M.J.S. Langman

Introduction to Clinical Examination
Second edition
Edited by John Macleod

An Introduction to Primary Medical Care
David Morrell

Urology and Renal Medicine
Second edition
J.B. Newsam and J.J.B. Petrie

Psychological Medicine for Students
John Pollitt

Respiratory Medicine
Malcolm Schonell

Cardiology for Students
Max Zoob